THE OLIVE OIL DIET

Dr Simon Poole and Judy Ridgway

ROBINSON

ROBINSON

First published in Great Britain in 2016 by Robinson

IMPORTANT NOTE
The recommendations in this book are solely intended as education
and information and should not be taken as medical advice.

A CIP catalogue record for this book
is available from the British Library.

ISBN: 978-1-47213-846-0

Typeset in New Caledonia by Hewer Text UK Ltd, Edinburgh
Printed and bound by CPI Group (UK) Ltd, Croydon, CR0 4YY

Papers used by Robinson are from well-managed forests and other responsible sources.

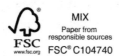

MIX
Paper from
responsible sources
FSC® C104740

Robinson
is an imprint of
Little, Brown Book Group
Carmelite House
50 Victoria Embankment
London EC4Y 0DZ

An Hachette UK Company
www.hachette.co.uk

www.littlebrown.co.uk

How To Books are published by Robinson, an imprint of Little, Brown Book
Group. We welcome proposals from authors who have first-hand experience
of their subjects. Please set out the aims of your book, its target market and
its suggested contents in an email to Nikki.Read@howtobooks.co.uk.

Dr Simon ⸻⸻⸻⸻⸻⸻⸻⸻⸻ ⸻l-time doctor in general practice in ⸻⸻⸻⸻⸻⸻⸻⸻⸻⸻ ⸻d international commentator on the Mediterranean Diet and is a member of the Council of Directors of the True Health Initiative in the USA. He has written regularly on matters related to primary care in medicine and nutrition for a diverse range of national media including the *Guardian, Nutrition and Food Science* and the *Journal of the Royal College of Surgeons* as well as consumer magazines such as *Cook Vegetarian* and *Body Language*. He also has extensive experience broadcasting and writing for local, national and international radio, television and web-based organisations. He regularly speaks at and chairs conferences attended by physicians, the media, politicians and the food industry on subject matters relating to health, politics and nutrition.

Judy Ridgway is an acclaimed food writer and international expert on olive oil. She was the first non-Italian judge to sit on the judging panel of the prestigious Leone d'Oro international awards for olive oil. She travels frequently to the producing regions, meeting the growers and tasting the oils along the way. She is also in regular contact with specialist cooking schools, university agricultural departments and research institutes. Previous books featuring olive oil include two editions of *Judy Ridgway's Best Olive Oil Buys Round the World, The Olive Oil Companion* and *Remarkable Recipes from the people who really know about extra virgin olive oil – the producers*. She has also written a number of other books on various aspects of food and wine, including *Food for Sport and Fitness* and *The Wine Tasting Class*, which was nominated for a Julia Child Award in America. She also has extensive experience of national TV and radio.

OTHER TITLES

CONTENTS

PREFACE

JUDY Ridgway and Simon Poole met in 2013 and immediately found that they had a strong mutual interest in olive oil. Judy is an acclaimed food writer and international expert on quality, taste and flavour in olive oil and Simon is a full-time GP who has also built up a vast body of knowledge of the nutrition and health benefits of olive oil. They were soon comparing notes and each found that the other's detailed knowledge dovetailed with their own to answer questions that had been occupying them both in recent years.

- Why is olive oil increasingly seen as a really healthy food?
- How does olive oil work in the body to protect against chronic diseases such as coronary disease and stroke?
- How can you find the healthiest olive oils?
- How much olive oil should we be consuming each day?
- What is the best way to include olive oil in everyday eating?

For some time, Simon had been monitoring the extensive, worldwide research which has established beyond doubt the health benefits of olive oil in the Mediterranean Diet and highlighted the many benefits that flow specifically from its regular use. Some of this research is reported in mainstream media, but much more frequently studies are published in journals of medicine, food chemistry or agriculture. This information is readily available to only a few, yet the sum total of this research has changed the thinking about olive oil in a major way. Simon believed that this information should have a wider audience.

Judy's work with olive growers and olive oil producers looking at the factors which lead to the production of top-quality olive oil was beginning to point to strong connections with the chemistry of the oil. The processes of cultivation, harvesting, production and storage all influence the quality of the finished oil and we now know that they also influence its capacity to have multiple beneficial effects on our well-being. It was also becoming evident that many of the substances which are responsible for the wonderful range of taste and flavour in olive oil were the very same chemicals which give olive oil its wide-ranging health benefits.

In addition, questions that Judy was receiving from readers and tasting class participants were focusing much more on the nutrition of olive oil than they had in the past. Health was becoming as important as the culinary aspects of olive oil. At the same time, Simon was discovering not only that olive oil is beneficial in its own right, but that the combination of olive oil with other ingredients to create good food also determines how people can optimise their health.

Hours of discussions and of sharing a passion for olive oil, good food and health resulted in the creation of the Olive Oil Diet. Judy and Simon both felt that there was a real need for a book which makes sense of the science **and** gives practical advice on incorporating olive oil into everyday eating, with practical hints, tips and recipes. *The Olive Oil Diet* does just this. It is designed to take the fear out of using significant amounts of olive oil in the diet. It also makes it easy to produce food which is broad ranging and enjoyable – and healthy at the same time.

IMPORTANT NOTE

The information included in this book reflects the current state of knowledge. It is based on research information published in journals and scientific articles which have been peer reviewed. Only information considered scientifically reliable has been used in compiling the evidence. The advice contained here is based on this evidence, often involving adult population studies. It should not replace the guidance or prescribed medications of a personal physician and in the event of allergies or special prescribed diets, further medical direction should be sought. Reference to this information should be made as a guide to making positive changes in diet and lifestyle. Regular exercise is also important to maintain a good state of health and fitness. If an individual has concerns about their capacity to make lifestyle changes they should seek further medical advice.

INTRODUCTION

THE Olive Oil Diet describes a diet for life. It is not a quick fix for losing weight. It is a way of living which has been shown to help people not only in achieving and maintaining a healthy weight but also in protecting them against chronic heart disease, strokes and much more. The extraordinary news is that after making changes like this, there are measurable improvements in a person's sense of well-being, quality of life and physical and mental health. To adopt the Olive Oil Diet is to commit to improved fitness, enjoyment and vitality for life – to really feel the difference!

Whilst we may not always be able to avoid chance events or genetic tendencies that will affect our life course, we now have a wealth of evidence to show that the right sort of food promotes healing, health and happiness. The science of nutrition is just scratching the surface of understanding the complex relationships between food and human health. There are no doubt many exciting discoveries yet to come. What is becoming increasingly clear is that we can only make sense of a truly healthy diet if we look at the whole diet and our broader lifestyle choices.

In the 1970s and 80s, at a time when low fat diets were being promoted in Western Europe, studies revealed that the healthiest lifestyle in the world could be found on the Greek island of Crete. What was not widely reported at the time was the fact that this was a diet high in fat – 35 to 40 per cent of calories came from fats. As much as 80 per cent of this fat came from a single ubiquitous food source which influenced the whole

1

diet – extra virgin olive oil. No single ingredient in any diet can be said to be so fundamental to the beneficial effect on health and longevity.

The science is extraordinary, and the database is constantly expanding. The EPIC Study of 40,000 Spaniards over more than a decade showed that the risk of death from heart disease was nearly halved in participants consuming a couple of tablespoons of olive oil a day. The same study showed that those who consumed the most olive oil had a decrease in death rates from any cause by an incredible 26 per cent.

The EPIC Study is a long study involving over half a million participants in ten European centres and it has been monitoring health in relation to diet for over 15 years. It has provided a great deal of information about diet and lifestyle, with subsets of populations looked at in terms of their use of specific foods, such as olive oil.

Another study based at the University of Bordeaux made headlines through its conclusions published in the Journal *Neurology* in 2011 that there was a 40 per cent reduction in the rate of strokes in the group of the 7,500 individuals who regularly consumed olive oil. The chances of developing other serious chronic diseases was also very significantly reduced, with the risk of developing type 2 diabetes halved with regular use of olive oil.

The Predimed (*Prevención con Dieta Mediterránea*) Study, based in Spain, has changed the way we look at the health benefits of extra virgin olive oil in the Mediterranean Diet. This was a well-designed, randomised, controlled study which involved over 7,000 participants at high risk of developing heart disease. Participants were randomly allocated into groups to receive a low-fat diet, a Mediterranean Diet supplemented with nuts or with high antioxidant extra virgin olive oil. The various subsets of this very large study continue to make headlines in subject areas as diverse as peripheral vascular disease, breast cancer and mental activity.

The outcome was quite extraordinary. The groups on the Mediterranean Diet supplemented with extra virgin olive oil and with nuts saw a 30 per cent reduction in rates of heart disease. The results were so convincing that the trial was stopped for ethical reasons before the planned end date because it was felt important to advise the group on the low-fat diet of the advantages that had become clearly demonstrable in the Mediterranean Diet groups.

As a result of this and other research, the European Union allows health claims on the benefits of olive oil, and in America the new US Dietary Guidelines Advisory Committee conclusions have ended the 40-year-long recommendation of a limit on total fat. It suggests instead that dietary advice should focus on optimising the best type of fat, and much current research points to olive oil as being that fat.

There are numerous other universities and study centres now looking in detail at the health effects of individual components of olive oil from the monounsaturated fat content to the many non-fatty acid components, such as vitamin E and polyphenol antioxidants, which may have an effect on the complex chemistry of our cells – for example, how they might prevent cancer cell growth, influence levels of cholesterol molecules or even affect the regulation of the DNA which expresses our genetic programming and determines ageing.

It is the aim of this book to make practical sense of this constantly expanding database of research so that everyone can understand how to enjoy olive oil at the heart of a healthy lifestyle. Olive oils are not all the same and the book also explores the effects of diverse varieties, growing techniques and production methods on the health characteristics of different olive oils, and points the way to those extra virgin oils which are likely to provide the most advantageous nutritional characteristics.

After decades of fast food, processed meals and the industrialisation of our eating habits, there is a quiet revolution occurring in many kitchens. Commentators and authors are questioning the safety of modern methods of food production and exposing the damaging consequences of rising levels of obesity and ill-health. As a result, we are beginning to see a return to a pattern of eating that uses fresh produce and is free from added sugars, salts and preservatives. The Olive Oil Diet goes even further, adding plenty of extra virgin olive oil to a rich variety of fresh fruit and vegetables, nuts and seeds, wholegrain cereals, fish and poultry. The combination can enhance the health qualities of all these ingredients.

- **Reduce blood pressure:** Combining olive oil with green salad vegetables rich in nitrates produces nitro fatty acids which can reduce blood pressure.
- **Reduce glycaemic load:** Eating olive oil with carbohydrate foods can decrease the absorption of sugar and so reduce the glycaemic load of a meal.
- **Preserve Omega-3:** Cooking fish in olive oil protects the heat-sensitive Omega-3 polyunsaturates in the fish from breaking down.
- **Improve nutrient absorption:** Cooking vegetables rich in fat-soluble vitamins with olive oil produces more beneficial, easily absorbable nutrients than if cooked separately.
- **Reduce harmful compounds:** Marinating meat in olive oil reduces the production of harmful compounds on cooking.

Using olive oil in this way is not new. Olive oil has been a central part of the culture of civilisations, both ancient and modern, in those regions where olive trees thrive, and its people have extolled the virtues of olive oil for centuries.

In compiling this book it has been fascinating to meet people who know and love olive oil, and to hear their stories, which resonate with our understanding of the science of olive oil. The intuitive knowledge of a Calabrian family whose organically grown, ancient variety of olive produces an extra virgin olive oil with a peppery vibrancy known for its health qualities, and the centenarian in Crete who wakes with a tumbler of local koroneiki olive oil, sips a robust red wine with lunch and retires to bed with a cup of tea infused with mountain herbs. These are traditions which have been passed down through the generations and reveal the vital role that olive oil plays at the heart of the Mediterranean way of life.

Today, modern research shows that there is a very strong scientific basis for claiming that the food known to the ancient Greeks as the 'gift of the gods' and dubbed by Homer as 'liquid gold' is indeed a super-food with massive nutritional health benefits.

PART 1

DISCOVERING THE SECRETS OF OLIVE OIL

OLIVE oil has, for many thousands of years, been a central part of the culture and lifestyle of the Mediterranean regions in which it is produced. It has always been regarded as an excellent cooking medium but also as a very healthy ingredient. In the middle of the twentieth century this reputation brought olive oil to northern Europe and to other non-producing areas. However, it has only been in recent years that modern research has begun to show that the reverence paid to olive oil in the past has a real scientific basis.

This emerging science is illustrated by the numerous published articles which describe the effects of components of olive oil that have a bearing on human health and the complex chemistry of our cells – for example, how they might prevent cancer cell growth, influence levels of cholesterol molecules or even affect the regulation of the DNA.

Research is also showing how the benefits to health of other ingredients, such as fruit and vegetables, are enhanced by using olive oil in the same dish. As a result of all this research there has been a major shift in advice regarding the amount of fat we should eat and the sort of fat that should be. Olive oil is taking over from seed oils as the preferred fat in the diet.

FAT THAT IS GOOD FOR YOU

F AT in our diet is essential. It is an important source of energy and it is necessary for many biochemical functions, such as the absorption of fat-soluble vitamins. Fat in our bodies helps to maintain healthy cell walls and plays a part in protecting and insulating our internal organs. It is important, too, in the regulation of body temperature and in keeping healthy hair and skin. Olive oil is a dietary fat which has even more benefits for us than other fats. The reason for this is its particular and unique composition.

Fat Has Had a Bad Press in Recent Years

Perhaps this is not surprising given the high level of calories in fat compared to proteins and carbohydrates and the pejorative use of the word 'fat' to describe the end result of the metabolic processes which dictates our body weight and appearance and contributes to our state of health.

Fat does contain a higher number of calories per gram than proteins and carbohydrates but not all fats have the same effect on weight and obesity. Monounsaturated fats, like oleic acid which is the predominant fat in olive oil, are not the same as other types of fat. For example, when oleic acid is absorbed and transported to the liver it is broken down in a different way from other fats. This makes it less likely to create excess body fat.

Indeed, monounsaturated fats may be less important in causing obesity than the glycaemic load or Glycaemic Index (GI) of carbohydrates in the diet. The Glycaemic Index measures the rise in blood sugar after eating. The risk of developing obesity and diabetes, in particular, are affected by the GI of foods. The rise in obesity levels in recent years is probably more related to the increase in high GI products – such as high-fructose corn syrup used in many processed products and sugary drinks – rather than in the consumption of fat.

Our bodies create fat to store the energy from excess, unutilised calories irrespective of where those calories originate. *Being overweight is not as simple as eating too much fat.*

Not only are there different types of fat that have very different implications for health, but the interactions between fats can also play an important part in how they affect our health. The wrong balance between these different fats can increase the risk of disease.

Fats in Our Food

Most dietary fats are made up of stable combinations of three individual types of fatty acid: polyunsaturated fatty acids, monounsaturated fatty acids and saturated fatty acids. These fatty acids are held together in a framework or chain of carbon molecules with hydrogen and oxygen. This framework is known as a glycerol and the whole structure is called a triglyceride.

There is also a fourth type of fatty acid called trans-fat which can occur in nature, but which is mainly produced artificially by the food-processing industry.

Polyunsaturated Fats
These have a chemical structure with two or more double bonds between the carbon atoms. There are two types of polyunsaturated fat

which are particularly important because they cannot be manufactured by the body itself. Thus they are known as essential fatty acids.

They are Omega-3 and Omega-6 and they perform different actions in the body. Their names refer to the position of the double bonds on the carbon chain. Omega-3 fats, the most common of which is alpha linolenic acid, have bonds in the third position. Omega-6 fats, the most common of which is linoleic acid, have bonds in the sixth position.

Polyunsaturated fats in the modern diet are predominantly found in vegetable oils, such as corn oil, sunflower oil and soya bean oil. Seeds are rich sources of Omega-6 and so the wide use of these seed oils means that we tend to consume quite large quantities of Omega-6. Oily fish, such as mackerel, tuna, salmon and sardines, are rich sources of Omega-3 but are consumed in considerably smaller quantities. There are also some plant sources of Omega-3, such as flax seed, some green vegetables and nuts.

Monounsaturated Fats

These fats, such as the oleic acid in olive oil, have only one double bond in their entire structure. Oleic acid is sometimes referred to as Omega-9, since its double bond is situated at the ninth carbon position in the fatty acid chain. Olive oil, rapeseed oil and avocado oil are all rich in monounsaturated fats.

Olive oil is made up mainly of monounsaturated fats, predominantly oleic acid, a fatty acid that takes its name from the olive. Proportions vary from 55 to 83 per cent with most olive oils having around 65 to 75 per cent oleic acid. Olive oil also contains significant amounts of Omega-6 polyunsaturated fat with traces of polyunsaturated linolenic acid. The remaining 10 to 18 per cent is made up of saturated fat. The wide range in these percentages is due to the large number of different olive varieties.

Saturated Fats

Saturated fats are defined by their lack of double bonds. All the carbon atoms have given up a bond to link with a hydrogen atom. Thus the fatty acid is 'saturated' or full up with hydrogen and so cannot carry any more. Most saturated fat in the diet comes from animal products, such as meat and dairy produce. The different saturated fatty acids vary in the degree to which they are absorbed by the body.

Trans-fats

Trans-fats are unsaturated fats which have undergone hydrogenation. This is a chemical process in which hydrogen is added to the original fat molecule. Unsaturated fats are not normally solid at room temperature. However, the hydrogenation process produces a hardened vegetable fat which is more easily used by the food industry.

Not So Simple Cholesterol

The proportion of different types of fat in our diet is important because it can influence the levels of cholesterol in the body. Cholesterol, like fat, has gained a reputation as a bad chemical, particularly when it comes to our risks of developing heart disease or having a stroke. However, the emerging understanding of the impact of cholesterol levels on the development of these conditions suggests that the link is much more complex than at first thought.

We need cholesterol in the body because it plays a significant role in the chemistry of our cells. It helps to keep the cell wall membranes well formed and strong. It also has a role carrying messages within the cell, including those that support the working of the nervous system.

Cholesterol is so essential that the body actually creates its own cholesterol in the liver. Cholesterol is attached to proteins to produce lipoproteins which are transported in the blood to cells around the body.

In fact, most cholesterol in the body is manufactured in the liver rather than being directly absorbed from our food and it is this home-grown cholesterol which represents most of the cholesterol in the blood.

We now know that not all forms of cholesterol are harmful. When the protein carrying cholesterol is in a so-called 'low-density' structure (low-density lipoprotein or LDL for short) there is an increased risk of heart disease or stroke, particularly if it is oxidised (see page 34). On the other hand if the protein carrying cholesterol is in a high-density structure (high-density lipoprotein or HDL), there is a beneficial effect and a reduced risk of these diseases.

In simple terms, LDL can cause the build-up of fatty plaques that narrow or block blood vessels which, particularly when inflamed, can result in catastrophic blood clots. HDL, the 'good' cholesterol, helps to reduce the levels of circulating cholesterol by returning it to the liver for recycling and so reduces the chances of diseased arteries.

Research has shown that the different types of fat in the diet can have quite different effects on levels of cholesterol in the blood. Saturated fats and trans-fats have been found to increase the levels of potentially harmful LDL whereas monounsatured and polyunsaturated fats are known to lower LDL. Monounsaturated fats may also increase levels of HDL. So having high levels of harmful cholesterol in the blood is not as simple as eating too much fat or cholesterol. It has much more to do with the type of fat that is eaten.

As a result of this understanding, the US Dietary Guidelines Committee has concluded that dietary cholesterol is not important and that foods such as eggs and prawns, which had previously been thought to be harmful due to their high levels of naturally occurring cholesterol, can be safely consumed in moderation.

One of the reasons that olive oil is considered to be such a healthy oil is that it is made up mainly of monounsaturated oleic acid, which has many beneficial effects in addition to its effect on cholesterol levels. For example, there is some evidence that oleic acid in olive oil increases insulin sensitivity, so improving sugar regulation and reducing the risk of develop-ing diabetes. This is true for all olive oil not just extra virgin olive oil.

Evolving Dietary Advice

Back in the 1960s and 1970s, the work of the Seven Countries Study by Professor Ancel Keys in America gained huge media coverage. The study showed much lower rates of heart disease in the southern Mediterranean countries than in northern Europe and North America. It also showed that similar differences were becoming apparent in those areas with changing patterns of consumption, moving from a traditional Mediterranean Diet high in unsaturated fats to a more northerly type of diet with higher levels of saturated fats.

The early conclusion drawn from these studies was that the best way to lower cholesterol levels and so reduce rates of heart disease was to replace saturated fats in the general diet with unsaturated fats. The most readily available unsaturated fats which could be produced in large quantities to make this replacement possible were polyunsatu-rated seed oils, which contain high levels of Omega-6 polyunsaturates.

Agriculture in the USA was able to produce these seed oils in abun-dance. Government subsidies coupled with public advertising campaigns encouraging people to increase their consumption of such oils set the scene for an exponential rise in their inclusion in processed foods and margarines.

This policy assumed that replacing saturated fats with polyunsatu-rated fats would have the same effects as those seen in the Mediterranean countries included in the studies. But the main source of fat in the Mediterranean Diet was monounsaturated fat from olive oil and not polyunsaturated fat.

Although it appears to be true that, when saturated fats are replaced by unsaturated fats, rates of heart disease decrease, researchers are questioning the different roles played by monounsaturated and polyunsaturated fats. Some scientists think that a diet high in polyunsaturated fats can be as harmful as a diet high in saturated fats. It may also depend on the proportions of the different types of fat.

Over the last two decades, many nutrition experts in the UK and in America, have favoured a low-fat, high-carbohydrate diet as the best way to avoid obesity and reduce heart disease. No indication was given about the type of fat or carbohydrate to be consumed. This advice, too, is now recognised as questionable. The wrong type of carbohydrate can increase the risk of obesity while conversely the right type of fat can improve health. The 2015 conclusions of the US Dietary Guidelines Advisory Committee have ended the 40-year-long recommendation of a limit on total fat. This statement will revolutionise dietary advice around the world: 'dietary advice should put the emphasis on optimising types of dietary fat and not reducing total fat'.

As more and more is understood about nutrition and health, the Mediterranean way of eating, with olive oil at its heart, is coming to be seen as an ideal diet for good health and long life. It has been shown time and again to reduce the risks of heart disease, stroke, many cancers and even dementia. It offers a pattern of eating which provides a natural combination of foods which we have evolved to eat. It is a 'whole' diet which transcends arguments over individual nutrients and which describes healthy ingredients to be included each day rather than foods to be avoided.

Unhealthy Ratios of Polyunsaturated Fats in our Diet

The high Omega-6 content of seed oils, now so widespread in the Western diet, has resulted in a ratio of approximately 16:1 of Omega-6 to Omega-3 polyunsaturates. This excess of Omega-6 fat has been shown to potentially have a pro-inflammatory effect (see page 28) and so may increase the risk of cardiovascular disease, precisely the reverse of what was intended by Western governments who were so keen to reduce our saturated fat consumption.

More natural diets tend towards more equal amounts of Omega-6 and Omega-3, with a ratio of less than 4:1. The Mediterranean Diet, using olive oil as the main source of fat, benefits from a high monounsaturated fat intake with a similarly balanced proportion of Omega-6 fats from meats, seeds and vegetables, and Omega-3 polyunsaturated fats derived from fish, nuts and other plant sources, such as green vegetables.

Sunflower and safflower seed oils have particularly high levels of Omega-6 and their success has contributed to the widening of the Omega-6 to Omega-3 ratio. To help reduce this wide gap a new generation of sunflower and safflower oils with lower levels of Omega-6 and higher level of Omega-9 oleic acid have been developed. However, these new oils do not have the antioxidant health benefits of extra virgin olive oil.

The balance of Omega-3 and Omega-6 polyunsaturates in olive oil itself varies depending on the individual olive oil. Extra virgin olive oils produced in more southerly regions of the Mediterranean frequently have rather higher levels of Omega-3 polyunsaturated fatty acids. This may relate to the low levels of rainfall, though there are no doubt other factors that have an influence. Some olive oils produced in the southern hemisphere have particularly high levels of Omega-3 polyunsaturated fat. However, the low relatively low levels of Omega-3 in olive oil are not significant in relation to the diet as a whole.

Not All Saturated Fats Are the Same

Although the general advice is to cut down on saturated fat because of the association between saturated fat in the diet and heart disease, not all saturated fats are as harmful as each other. Fatty acids differ in the length of the molecular chain making up their carbon 'backbone'. They may have a small, medium or long molecular chain. Some long-chain fatty acids, such as palmitic acid found in meat and cow's milk dairy products, are more unhealthy because they are particularly associated with rises in potentially harmful LDL cholesterol. However, others, like stearic acid found in dark chocolate, do not adversely affect cholesterol.

Cheese made from free-range goat's milk or ewes' milk rather than cows' milk is commonly eaten in the Mediterranean region. It seems that the medium-chain saturated fats in these dairy products may be less harmful than the long-chain saturated fats found in higher concentrations in hard cheeses made from cows reared on a diet of grains.

In the same way that there are differences between the saturated fats in different cheeses so there are differences in the saturated fats found in olive oil and other monounsaturated oils. These distinctions are important because comparisons of levels of saturated fat are not as simple as they first appear.

It is also becoming apparent that individual types of saturated fats found in meat or dairy products have subtle chemical differences from vegetable sources of saturated fats. These variations can have very different effects in the body.

Summary

1 Being overweight is not as simple as eating too much fat.

2 There are three types of fat predominant in our diet: saturated, monunsaturated and polyunsaturated. Olive oil is made up predominantly of monounsaturated fat.

3 The proportion of different types of fat in our diet is important because it influences levels of cholesterol in the blood.

4 It is not eating cholesterol in the diet which causes problems but eating the wrong sort of fat.

5 Monounsaturated fat lowers levels of harmful LDL and may raise levels of beneficial HDL cholesterol.

6 When unsaturated fat replaces saturated fat in the diet heart disease rates are reduced. However, there is a debate about the effects of different ratios of polyunsaturated and monounsaturated fats.

7 Current advice includes recommending a Mediterranean Diet based on olive oil as the main source of fat.

8 A ratio of Omega-6 to Omega-3 of 4:1 is probably better than a diet with a very high level of Omega-6 polyunsaturated fats.

9 Not all saturated fat is the same. Some types are not as detrimental to our bodies as others.

HEART-HEALTHY ANTIOXIDANTS

EXTRA virgin olive oil is made up predominantly of fatty acids but it also contains around 1.5 to 2 per cent non-fatty acid constituents, such as vitamins, polyphenols, colour pigments and volatile components which contribute to the smell and taste of the oil. Indeed, more than 200 different chemicals have been identified in extra virgin olive oil. It now seems that these constituents are even more influential than its healthy fat content in maintaining good health and decreasing the risk of disease.

The Power of Antioxidants

Substances such as the tyrosol group of compounds, which are among the non-fatty acid chemicals found in extra virgin olive oil, are attracting intense interest from scientists seeking to unlock the secrets of olive oil. These compounds are part of a group of biochemical components known as phenolic antioxidants or polyphenols. The way in which they act in the body is one of the keys to fully understanding the health benefits of olive oil. These same chemicals are also important for their contribution to the basic taste characteristics of olive oil and to its quality and longevity (see page 88).

For some time it has been officially accepted that olive oil has a beneficial effect on health but the reasons for this were not entirely clear. In

2004 the Food and Drugs Administration in the USA allowed producers to promote the advantage of replacing saturated fats in the diet with two tablespoons of monounsaturated fat in the form of olive oil. However, we now know that it is not just the type of fat that is important in terms of health but that the non-fatty acid components in extra virgin olive oil, of which antioxidants are a significant element, are equally important.

In 2012 the European Food Safety Authority (EFSA) accepted that this was indeed the case. Whilst tightening regulations around food health labelling claims and scrutinising over 3,000 health claim submissions, EFSA permitted a health claim for those olive oils which contain a minimum concentration of phenolic antioxidants (see page 24).

'Polywhatsits' – So What Are Phenolic Antioxidants?

The cells of our bodies are in a constant state of chemical flux at a molecular and atomic level. This multitude of chemical reactions is necessary for every aspect of living and is the means by which we breathe, move, think and repair our bodies. They are fundamental to life and continue even when we are asleep.

However, many of these reactions have the potential to produce unstable by-products called free radicals. These free radicals have the capacity to damage the cells of the body in a process called oxidative stress and this can lead to a variety of diseases (see page 20). The best way to understand this is to compare these cellular reactions to billions of tiny nuclear reactors which produce energy, but which can also producer highly reactive waste.

Antioxidants are naturally occurring molecules in our food which can neutralise or mop up the free radicals and so repair the damage done through oxidative stress and help to keep the body in a healthy state. Many polyphenols have this antioxidant capacity. One such group of polyphenols – tyrosol and related compounds – is uniquely abundant in olive oil. It is measurably powerful in preventing the oxidation of cholesterol (see page 29), considered to be a key step in the development of heart disease.

Free Radicals, Oxidative Stress Theory and Antioxidants

Free Radicals

All of the structures in our bodies are made up of molecules which consist of atoms joined together in particular patterns. Each atom is a little like our solar system with a central positively charged core called a nucleus, surrounded by circulating negatively charged pairs of electrons. The pairing of these negatively charged electrons orbiting around the positively charged nucleus makes the atom stable.

The constant chemical reactions which occur in all living creatures inevitably creates by-products of atoms which have lost an electron from a pair. These atoms are unstable and some will 'scavenge' electrons from other atoms in the molecules of our cellular structures.

This in turn will destabilise the 'scavenged' atoms and a chain reaction will be set off, where unstable atoms with unpaired electrons will go on to further disrupt other atoms in our cells, causing damage and the potential for disease. These unstable atoms – called free radicals – can create a whirlwind of damaging chemical reactions in our bodies unless their demand for electrons and stability can be stopped.

Oxidative Stress

The process of free radicals with unpaired electrons stealing an electron from another atom is called 'oxidation'. The word comes from the observation that a very common atom which is necessary for living, oxygen, is a particularly strong scavenger of electrons when it has unpaired electrons. The powerful effects of oxygen can be seen when iron rusts, apples turn brown and fats become rancid. These unstable forms of oxygen are called 'reactive oxygen species'.

Other atoms can also damage our cells, for example unstable forms of nitrogen or 'reactive nitrogen species'. Where our bodies are at risk from oxidation by free radicals such as these, we are said to be subjected to 'oxidative stress' which causes damage to cells and makes us vulnerable to diseases and chronic inflammation (see page 28).

Antioxidants

Although we have internal systems to try to neutralise the oxidative damage that can be wreaked upon cells by free radicals, we rely on nutrients in our food which have the capacity to donate electrons to stabilise these reactive species.

There are many of these naturally occurring molecules, called anti-oxidants, particularly in fruits and vegetables. Many are the result of plants having evolved to ensure their fruits are themselves protected from the damaging oxidative stress in their environment. Many foods which have been described as 'superfoods' have antioxidants in abundance, and have been shown to protect us from chronic diseases.

External factors, such as smoking and pollutants, can also increase the number of free radicals in the body with the potential to cause harm. This can be due to increased exposure to damaging oxidation or to a decrease in antioxidant capacity within the body through detrimental lifestyle patterns coupled with bad diet.

It would be wrong, however, to characterise a healthy state as being devoid of all possible oxidative stress. The inevitable presence of free radicals has resulted in an evolutionary response to create a balanced state of 'redox' in our cells where the oxidative stress is balanced by the natural antioxidant capacity of our cells. This, with an adequate intake of antioxidants in our diet, enables our bodies to successfully manage the potentially harmful by-products of internal chemical reactions or external pollutants.

There is also evidence that the presence of a low concentration of reactive molecules may have some beneficial effects, including defence against attack by infections and supporting the immune system. When we exercise, there is an inevitable increase in intensity of chemical activity in our bodies, and it is our natural response to balance this to achieve the 'redox' state. The end result of this is that exercise is good for us!

Antioxidant Supplements – A Word of Warning

When the potential benefit of antioxidants in our diet was first discovered, there was considerable hope that simply taking supplements of naturally occurring antioxidants would decrease susceptibility to illness, or even cure existing disease.

Concentrated forms of many antioxidants are on sale in many shops and online. From vitamin E capsules, extracts of blueberries or concentrated garlic tablets – the variety and cost is very variable, and the health claims equally diverse. There is even a supplement of olive tree leaf extract.

However, despite the theories and the confident assertions made by manufacturers, scientific studies have failed to show any convincing benefit from artificial supplementation in this context. Indeed there have been studies which show that certain supplements can be harmful. Although population studies suggest that diets high in vitamin E and beta carotene are associated with a reduced risk of lung cancer, when vitamin E and carotene supplements were given to patients who were suffering from lung cancer, the survival rates of those taking the additional artificial antioxidant were actually lowered.

One possible explanation for this outcome may lie in the balanced state of 'redox' that is found in our cells (see page 22). The balance of free radicals and the antioxidant capacity required to keep our bodies in a healthy state is subtle and can be adversely affected by artificially high levels of supplemented antioxidants. This may discourage the need for our cells to produce natural antioxidant defences or utilise appropriately the many and varied forms of chemicals we find in a normal, healthy diet.

The interactions between compounds in foods and the way in which we absorb them and use them are more complex than throwing a bundle of antioxidants into the diet in the hope that this will protect us. There are other factors involved. For example, some minerals, including selenium and zinc, play a vital role in the processes by which free radicals are neutralised.

Antioxidants in Olive Oil

The most important group of antioxidants present in extra virgin olive oil are polyphenols. The most significant of these are those derived from tyrosol; tyrosol itself and hydroxytyrosol, oleuropein and a number of other compounds. Extra virgin olive oil also contains other types of polyphenols, such as lignans, flavonols and anthocyanins.

Numerous studies have been undertaken describing the effects of phenolic antioxidants on the body and the benefits have been shown to be many and varied. Their activity in neutralising damaging free radicals (see page 20) is a function which prevents many chronic degenerative conditions. They also protect us from developing circulatory disorders, such as heart problems and strokes, and may help to prevent the growth of cancers. They have been shown to support healthy bone formation and beneficially affect cholesterol levels. They help to decrease levels of chemicals which are associated with inflammation and also have antimicrobial activity.

The list of benefits grows as more research comes through. A recent study from the University of Louisiana proposes a mechanism by which olive oil polyphenols might lessen the oxidative stress which may be a cause of Alzheimer's dementia. Interestingly this condition is less prevalent in countries with a Mediterranean lifestyle.

Phenolic antioxidants are only found in extra virgin and virgin olive oils. The refining process strips out the vast majority of the non-fatty acid components. However, some vitamin E remains and this does have antioxidant properties of its own, which contribute to the health benefits of all types of olive oil.

Levels of polyphenols in extra virgin olive oil can vary from less than 50mg/kg to 700mg/kg. Most oils which are mass produced in large-scale units are thought to vary around average levels of approximately 200mg/kg. Premium oils, which are usually produced in smaller batches, are more likely to have higher levels at 300mg/kg to 550mg/kg.

Whilst absolute levels of polyphenols vary between extra virgin olive oils, the proportion of tyrosol remains remarkably constant in relation to the other less abundant polyphenols. They outnumber the other polyphenol groups by average ratios of 25–400:1. It is difficult to accurately measure the individual polyphenols, particularly if they are only present in small quantities, and there is a good deal of debate about the viability of the different methods of analysis. However, the fact that the tyrosol group of polyphenols is so universally dominant is very important in relation to the measurement of polyphenol content when making health claims.

European Food Safety Authority Scrutinises Olive Oil Antioxidants

The European Food Safety Authority (EFSA) is an independent agency which advises European countries on matters relating to food safety and regulation. Each country has the power to enforce the EFSA guidance to ensure compliance.

Until recently there was a very random approach to health claims made by food producers, but in 2014 a much more consistent protocol was instigated and the process of submitting a claim for appraisal by the committee became very rigorous. The outcome of the analysis of the research to support each application determines whether or not food producers can label an ingredient in terms of any health benefit. As a result of this, many food producers have been required to remove unfounded health claims from their packaging.

In recent years, EFSA has evaluated a number of studies which show the antioxidant effect of polyphenols in extra virgin olive oil in powerfully protecting the body from oxidation of LDL cholesterol (see page 19). As a result, EFSA has stated that a cause-and-effect relationship has been established between the consumption of polyphenols in extra virgin olive oil and the protection of LDL cholesterol from oxidative damage, and that the polyphenol content of an extra virgin oil should be measured by its levels of hydroxytyrosol and its derivatives. In its report EFSA states:

'The panel considers that in order to bear the claim, 5mg of hydroxytyrosol and its derivatives in olive oil should be consumed daily. These amounts, if provided by moderate amounts of olive oil, can be easily consumed in the context of a balanced diet. The concentrations in some oils may be too low to allow consumption of this amount of polyphenols in the context of a balanced diet.'

Given what we know about the proportional quantities of tyrosols in extra virgin olive oils, this desired level of consumption can be achieved with two tablespoons per day of oils which have total polyphenol levels of 250mg/kg or more.

In recognising the capacity of olive oil to protect LDL cholesterol from oxidative damage, EFSA has uniquely identified olive oil as playing an important role in the prevention of chronic disease. In addition, the research data which was analysed by the committee included several studies that demonstrated a proportional relationship between low, moderate and high levels of polyphenol antioxidants with an increase in therapeutic effect.

This has great significance as it recognises that there is a difference in health benefits between different olive oils. The concentrations of polyphenols in some olive oils are too low to satisfy the consumption required in the context of a balanced diet.

Summary

1 It is not just the type of fat in the diet that is important to health, but also the level of phenolic antioxidants in that fat.

2 Antioxidants work by mopping up and stabilising harmful free radicals, which are produced as a result of the ongoing biochemical activity in the body.

3 Antioxidants also help to keep the cells of the body in a balanced state of equilibrium and therefore in a healthy condition. When this equilibrium is disturbed, the work of the cells is disrupted and this can lead to a greater tendency towards diseases of various kinds.

4 Taking antioxidant supplements does not have the same effect as consuming natural antioxidants in food.

5 There are a number of powerful antioxidants in extra virgin olive oil and their activity has been shown to include many health

benefits, including their protective role in coronary heart disease.

6 Now the European Food Safety Agency has also approved health claims for extra virgin olive oils with a polyphenol content of more than 250mg/kg. The advice is to consume two to three tablespoon of such oils per day.

THE MEDICINAL FRUIT JUICE

THE importance of olive oil in the diet does not just rest on its protective role against coronary heart disease nor in its ability to reduce oxidative stress. It also has important anti-inflammatory properties. Inflammation is a process associated with many chronic illnesses and diseases. Infections and arthritis are obvious examples of inflammatory condition, but inflammation is not simply a result of bacterial attack or a risk to joints, it is also a general marker of other diseases and conditions.

Beneficial Inflammation

Inflammation is a series of processes by which our bodies protect us from acute illness or injury. The mobilisation of our immune system to isolate and deal with harmful attacks from an infection produces a response designed to destroy invading bacteria or viruses.

This response includes the production of powerful chemicals including free radicals (see page 20) which attack these unwanted infective agents. They also increase blood flow, temperature and swelling in the area. In acute illness this inflammation is followed by healing and repair to cells once the cause has been removed and the body returns to normal.

Chronic Inflammation

Inflammation can also occur in chronic illnesses which are not the result of infection and the results can be harmful. The body's immune system may be triggered to respond to damage in this way by external factors, such as smoking, UV light and toxins and chemical pollutants in the environment or by the production of free radicals and subsequent oxidative stress from chemical reactions in the body.

This kind of inflammation can have long-term harmful effects on our health. A vicious circle can be set up with the immune system attempting to protect cells from damage, yet paradoxically also contributing to the problem. Inflammation produces more free radicals in the body, which in turn lead to further oxidative stress and, if not stopped, to yet more free radicals and more inflammation and so on. This process, in time, will lead to chronic illness.

The link between free radicals, oxidative stress and harmful inflammation means that diets high in antioxidants can reduce inflammation by neutralising free radicals and so reducing the oxidative stress. On the other hand foods such as trans-fats, some polyunsaturated fats and some sugars can promote the likelihood of its development. Thus particular foods may be inflammatory or anti-inflammatory.

Clogs and Clots

Heart disease, for example, is a condition characterised by chronic inflammation. The most common forms of chronic disease – coronary heart disease and strokes – are usually the result of clogged arteries, which dangerously reduce blood supply to the heart, brain and other organs. This narrowing of the arteries is caused by a process known as 'arteriosclerosis'.

If the body produces high levels of cholesterol in the form of LDL, perhaps as a result of poor diet, free radical oxidation of this LDL may occur, creating unstable molecules which penetrate the lining of red blood vessels and set up an inflammatory response. The natural response to inflammation is to confine and seal off the damaged area and the blood vessel wall builds up to form a plaque. This, in turn, results in a narrowing and possible blockage of the artery.

To lessen the risk of haemorrhage through an injured or breached blood vessel, there is also an increased tendency to form blood clots. With further oxidative stress, these blood clots can break off and enter the circulation, causing sudden and catastrophic loss of blood to vital organs. This is what occurs during an acute heart attack or a stroke.

Although the accumulation of arteriosclerosis plaque occurs over many years, there are numerous studies which show that the addition of olive oil to the diet can reduce the risk of acute events, even if the diet is adopted in later life. This appears to confirm that olive oil can prevent the acute episodes of oxidation that lead to plaque rupture and clots, as well as preventing blood vessel disease over the long term. This is not only the case in the blood vessels which supply the heart, but also in blood vessels which go to other parts of the body – the so-called peripheral vascular system.

A subset of the Predimed study showed that rates of peripheral vascular disease (PVD) were reduced by more than two-thirds in people who adopted a Mediterranean Diet supplemented with high-antioxidant extra virgin olive oil. Researchers in the same study also found that irregular heart beat (atrial fibrillation), another risk factor for dangerous blood clots, was reduced by 38 per cent.

Extra Virgin Olive Oil as an Anti-inflammatory

However, there are other reasons why foods such as extra virgin olive oil can influence inflammation. Some polyphenols have the capacity to act on the inflammation itself in chemical processes which are separate from the process of oxidation. For example, some polyphenols in extra virgin olive oil have been shown to affect levels of detrimental enzymes found in arthritic joints and thus decrease inflammation. Studies using refined olive oils did not show these effects. Research has also confirmed that patients with rheumatoid arthritis who were given additional extra virgin olive oil in their diet described lower levels of pain, swelling and joint symptoms.

One phenol in extra virgin olive oil has received particular attention for its anti-inflammatory effects. This compound is called oleocanthal ('oleo' meaning olive and 'canth' meaning sting). The remarkable story of its discovery in 2005 is a serendipitous tale of science and food.

A new over-the-counter cold remedy had been introduced to the market by a American pharmaceutical company, but consumer feedback had suggested that one of its components produced a harmless but rather strong irritant sensation on the throat. The producers asked the Monell Chemical Senses Institute in Philadelphia to investigate. The Institute knew that one of the ingredients in the remedy was ibuprofen, so they set to work to understand the mechanism by which this anti-inflammatory caused this minor cough when in liquid form.

Coincidentally, one of the scientists from Monell, Gary Beauchamp, was travelling to Italy where he sampled some fresh extra virgin olive oil. He noticed a very similar, mild irritant effect, which occasionally resulted in the same distinctive cough. This led to research at Monell which showed that although ibuprofen and oleocanthal in extra virgin olive oil are chemically quite distinct, they have a similar effect on our taste sensations and share anti-inflammatory properties.

It has been estimated that 50ml of extra virgin olive oil rich in oleocanthal polyphenols may provide an equivalent anti-inflammatory effect to 200mg of ibuprofen. Similarly, the presence of this and other natural anti-inflammatories in extra virgin olive oil may contribute to the lower rates of arthritis, asthma, inflammatory bowel diseases and other chronic diseases.

The causes of the joint inflammation in osteoarthritis are different to those of rheumatoid arthritis. It is a condition which is based on wear and tear and resultant bone thinning rather than on an individual's own immune system contributing to the destruction of a normal joint. In this connection, scientists have discovered the importance of a substance called lubricin, which protects normal joints. Lubricin is reduced in inflamed osteoarthritic joints, but it can be restored and inflammation reduced through regular exercise and a diet rich in extra virgin olive oil. In addition, the regular consumption of olive oil has been shown to increase the absorption of minerals such as calcium and promote the capacity of the body to use them to form the rigid structures in bone.

Ulcerative colitis is another inflammatory condition which causes pain, bleeding and other complications. Research at the University of East Anglia has shown that the oleic acid in olive oil seems to help prevent the development of the disease by blocking chemicals in the bowel that aggravate the inflammation.

Extra Virgin Olive Oil and Cancer

For many years, scientists have observed lower rates of many different types of cancer in people who most closely follow a Mediterranean Diet rich in olive oil. Studies are now showing specific links with extra virgin olive oil. The antioxidant and anti-inflammatory effects of the regular consumption of good-quality extra virgin olive oil help to avert the damaging effects of oxidation which can lead to cell and DNA damage, which in turn can cause cancerous changes as the genetic programming of cells is disrupted.

Individual studies associating reduced cancer risk with extra virgin olive oil are published with increasing frequency, but even more powerful and exciting conclusions can be drawn from studies of studies – so-called systematic review 'meta analyses'. This process is where researchers combine the work of several published studies to analyse the combined results.

In 2010 and 2011, research centres in Milan and Athens released meta analyses providing convincing evidence describing the relationship between consuming extra virgin olive oil and lower risks of a number of cancers. These included cancer of the breast, respiratory tract and gastrointestinal tract, including cancer of the oesophagus and colon.

In separate studies it has been shown that there may be a reduction in rates of progression of breast cancer and some skin cancers with a higher consumption of extra virgin olive oil. Indeed a small sub-group within the Spanish Predimed study (see page 2) were found to have a 68 per cent reduction of risk of breast cancer. Interestingly, it has been found that there are some chemical similarities between lignans in extra virgin olive oil and tamoxifen, which is used to treat and some-times to prevent breast cancer. Some research suggests that the oleic acid in olive oil might work with anti-cancer drugs to enhance their benefit. Many scientists are now focusing on the ability of components in olive oil to control and regulate those genes in our cells, 'turning on' protective genes.

Reports from research with small groups following a Mediterranean Diet enriched with olive oil in Switzerland, Italy and New Zealand also show encouraging results in relation to reduced risk for cancer of the womb and a reduced risk of progression of prostate cancer in men.

Olive Oil and High Blood Pressure

High blood pressure combines with oxidised cholesterol on blood vessel walls to increase the risk of heart disease and strokes. Factors in extra virgin olive oil have been shown not only to benefit cholesterol levels and reduce its oxidation, but also to lower blood pressure.

There has been some fascinating recent research which has shown that combining the monounsaturated fatty acids of olive oil with the nitrate compounds commonly found in salads, green salad leaves and vegetables produces nitro fatty acids. These nitro fatty acids act to keep blood pressure low.

Not only can a diet rich in olive oil prevent high blood pressure, it has also been shown that if people already taking medication for high blood pressure adopt such a diet, their blood pressure can fall signifi-cantly and their need for medication be reduced.

Food for Thought – Strokes, Dementia, Alzheimer's and Parkinson's Disease

Strokes are usually the result of clogs and clots in blood vessels which supply oxygen and nutrients to the brain. A stroke can have a devastating effect and cause paralysis and even death. The same factors that affect the blood vessels of the heart (see page 29) have similar influences on blood vessels elsewhere. The effects of good fats and polyphenol antioxidants on reducing the damaging effects of oxidation of cholesterol will protect the integrity and function of the blood vessels to the brain.

In 2011 the respected journal *Neurology* published a paper from a group of researchers from Bordeaux University studying 7,500 individuals. They observed that on average those who were consuming more olive oil had a reduced risk of stroke of 41 per cent. The difference in percentage risk of stroke between those who reported the greatest daily use of olive oil and those with the lowest consumption was an extraordinary 78 per cent.

As part of the Predimed Study (see page 2), researchers undertook ultrasound scans of the major blood vessels leading to the brains of the participants and measured the sizes of the plaques that were present. The findings concluded that the diet enriched with extra virgin olive oil resulted in significantly slower progression of these plaques.

Some common forms of dementia are the result of multiple tiny strokes affecting intellectual functioning. This vascular dementia is less common in regions where extra virgin olive oil is used as part of the Mediterranean Diet. Given what we know about the beneficial effects of extra virgin olive oil on blood vessels large and small, this is entirely consistent with what might be expected.

Alzheimer's Disease, which is another common form of dementia, is also reduced in people who follow a Mediterranean Diet. Unlike vascular dementia, the underlying cause of Alzheimer's Disease is not well understood. A popular theory is that oxidative stress is a precursor of the production of abnormal proteins which form in a particular pattern in the brain. It is possible that the antioxidant properties of substances like oleocanthal and oleuropein in extra virgin olive oil may protect the brain from the illness.

Although Parkinson's Disease is a distinct neurological condition, it shares with Alzheimer's Disease the common factor of cell death in the brain leading to loss of function. Although this can involve intellectual function, the first symptom is usually loss of movement control. A major review of published data on the Mediterranean Diet by Dr Sofi at the University of Florence observed a 13 per cent reduced rate of Parkinson's Disease in people who follow such a diet. Some researchers believe that vitamin E, present in high quantities in extra virgin olive oil, may contribute to that protective effect, though more recently oleocanthal has also been considered to play a part.

The causes of Parkinson's Disease are not yet fully understood, but it is clear that brain cells are particularly susceptible to oxidative stress, and it is very likely that the unique proportions of antioxidants in extra virgin olive oil may play a significant role in protecting our mental health in older age.

Yet More Benefits

In addition to phenolic antioxidants and anti-inflammatories, extra virgin olive oil contains a number of other important chemicals, such as vitamin E and squalene, which contribute to its health benefits. Many of these constituents have yet to be fully investigated.

Vitamin E, or tocopherol, is present in both extra virgin olive oil and in refined olive oil. However, the refining process removes a proportion of the vitamin from the oil. Vitamin E has antioxidant effects and can also reduce the likelihood of blood clots by limiting the aggregation of platelets – the blood cells that are in part responsible for the formation of clots. It may also play a role in preventing the formation of plaques which lead to heart disease and strokes. Deficiency of vitamin E has also been associated with an increased risk of cancers of the lung, cervix and prostate.

The distinctive aromas and flavours of olive oil come from a range of hydrocarbons including hexanals. These compounds have been shown to possess antimicrobial effects, which may protect us from bacteria, such as *E. coli* and *Staphylococcus*. Studies of these chemicals are at an early stage, but show that the taste properties of an oil might also contribute further to our health.

Research in Germany has led to the suggestion that the inclusion of olive oil in a meal can lead to higher levels of satiety and measurably increased levels of serotonin – a hormone associated with fullness. Even the scent of olive oil on our food may create a sense of satisfaction through the meal, which allows us to eat less and to better manage the effect of the foods that we consume. The compound which was used in the research to impart the aroma of olive oil was hexanal. This is known to be the scent which gives the 'grassy' characteristic to some extra virgin olive oils.

Squalene is another hydrocarbon found in many plant foods but the concentrations in extra virgin olive oil are uniquely high. In refined oils they are rather lower. Squalene is a powerful antioxidant and some scientists believe that much of the observed decrease in rates of cancers of the breast, pancreas and colon associated with higher intake of olive oil may be in part due the high levels of squalene in the oil. In addition, squalene is often found in high concentrations in the skin of people who consume olive oil regularly. Its antioxidant activity has been shown to inhibit the formation of skin cancers.

Squalene is also found in the body. It is one of the intermediate molecules produced in the formation of natural cholesterol. However, its regular consumption does not appear to raise levels of cholesterol in the blood. On the contrary, studies show that taking a supplement of squalene alongside the cholesterol-lowering statin drug, pravastatin, enhances the beneficial effect of the medication.

Summary

1 Inflammation is a factor in infections and injuries and in many chronic illnesses and diseases, such as heart disease, strokes, arthritis, asthma, ulcerative colitis and cancer.

2 Oxidative stress caused by the action of free radicals can lead to inflammation.

3 Phenolic antioxidants in extra virgin olive oil can reduce oxidative stress and so help to reduce inflammation.

4 There are other polyphenols in extra virgin olive oil which can combat inflammation itself. One of these is oleocanthal, which works in a similar way to the chemical ibuprofen.

5 In addition to antioxidants and anti-inflammatories, extra virgin olive oil also contains other beneficial chemicals, such as vitamin E and squalene.

6 Extra virgin olive oil is a healthy cocktail of numerous naturally occurring chemicals which combine to reduce the risk of a range of chronic diseases.

KEEPING A HEALTHY WEIGHT –
THE END OF DIETING?

W E have come to think of diets as ways of fighting the growing obesity epidemic in the Western world. Diets usually involve restricting what we can eat. For many, being on a diet, means 'Dare I eat that?' Dieting is often a recipe for misery. Yet research shows that many people have tried numerous different diets in their life-time, and most have failed to sustain any long-term weight loss or health benefits.

If we view diets simply as eating to lose weight, even if this is success-ful, it is questionable how valuable this might be unless we are able to be sure this is a more healthy state. The Olive Oil Diet which is described in this book reflects the original meaning of the word 'diet' which derives from the Greek word *diatia* which describes a way of life. In ancient Greek culture, this extended beyond food to physical fitness and how to live well as an individual in society. As we wrestle with the ethical and quality issues of intensive farming techniques, the effects of food production on our environment, fast food and the way supply is driven by commercial priorities, perhaps we can learn more from viewing a diet as a way of life.

Not All Calories Are the Same

Olive oil is a fat and contains approximately 120 calories per table-spoon. In a culture where we have been frequently advised to count and limit our calories, this is enough to put many people off the regular use of olive oil.

However, there is no evidence that regular consumption of olive oil causes weight gain or is particularly likely to result in obesity. On the contrary, numerous studies show that following a diet that includes unrestricted amounts of olive oil, such as the Mediterranean Diet, is very much consistent with maintaining a healthy weight. This way of eating has also been shown to protect people at risk of developing type 2 diabetes, which is often associated with being overweight.

Other studies show that consuming olive oil has a protective effect against coronary heart disease, raised blood pressure, certain cancers and a range of other chronic conditions, so it would hardly make sense if olive oil was guilty of piling on the weight. After all, increasing obesity is associated with the very conditions from which olive oil can help to protect us.

The answer to this seeming contradiction lies in a greater understanding not only of calories and how they work in the body but also of the roles and interactions between different foods in the overall pattern of eating. This is not as simple as is sometimes portrayed. Our bodies do not just add up the calorific value of the food we eat minus the amount of energy we burn in our activities, and add the difference in calories to our waists or hips!

All fats have the same calorie content but different fats have a different tendency to result in weight gain. The monounsaturated oleic fat in olive oil appears to contribute much less to the fat we accumulate than other types of fat, such as saturated fats. When oleic acid is absorbed, the ways in which it is transported and then broken down by the liver for use by the body is different from the processes undergone by other fats. This makes it less likely that oleic acid will end up causing the laying down of excess body fat.

We also now know that excess energy from high glycaemic index carbohydrates, such as sugar and refined and processed grains, is a more important risk factor for weight gain. This is despite the fact that high-sugar drinks, for example, contain relatively few calories per 100g compared with other foods, such as olive oil and whole grains.

Extra Virgin Olive Oil and Glycaemic Index

When carbohydrate food is eaten it is broken down in the gut into sugars, which are then absorbed into the body via the blood system in the form of glucose to provide energy. The body naturally regulates blood glucose levels by producing a hormone called insulin. This is the hormone which allows us to store the energy available from sugars in our diet in the form of fat for use when we need it.

Different foods break down, and so raise blood sugar levels, more quickly than others. The speed at which this happens is known as the glycaemic index (GI) of the food. Simple carbohydrates, such as refined sugar, have a high glycaemic rating as they break down quickly and result in a rapid build-up of glucose in the blood. Complex carbo-hydrates, such as whole grains, on the other hand, take much longer to break down into glucose and so have a low glycaemic rating.

Most modern diets include many high-glycaemic index foods made with refined grains and sugars and often with added sweeteners, like high fructose corn syrup or glucose syrup. Such a diet is likely to result in high blood-sugar levels and associated risks of weight gain, obesity and ultimately type 2 diabetes.

Although olive oil itself effectively has no glycaemic index because it contains negligible amounts of carbohydrate, it can have an effect on other foods that do. In common with some acidic foods, such as lemon juice and vinegar, olive oil can influence the breakdown of starchy carbohydrates in a meal and slow down the rise in sugars from the other ingredients.

It is useful to know the glycaemic index of a particular food, but it is important to understand that this may be affected by how it is cooked and prepared – and more specifically, if the food is consumed with a generous drizzle of extra virgin olive oil!

Extra Virgin Olive Oil Affects Insulin Sensitivity

Insulin ensures that blood glucose levels are kept within a certain safe and effective range for the body. Very high levels of glucose in the blood can be toxic and damaging, so the right amount of insulin produced, for example, after a meal will ensure that excess glucose is taken for storage in the liver, muscle and fat cells where it will be available when it is needed for energy.

Most healthy people have what is known as 'high insulin sensitivity', which means that only small amounts of the hormone are required to adequately control rises in blood sugars. This is particularly the case if the sugars in the diet are mainly in the form of complex carbohydrates which are broken down over a longer period of time, meaning that the rise in blood sugars after a meal is slow.

Those who need more insulin to do the same job are described as having 'low insulin sensitivity' or being 'insulin resistant'. This can happen when we are ill or at times of stress or it may be the result of long-term exposure to foods with a high glycaemic index and the consequent weight gain. Some people have an in-built deficiency in making adequate amounts of insulin. Type 1 diabetes is an example where there is not enough insulin manufactured to meet the body's need to regulate glucose levels.

The exact mechanisms for developing insulin resistance and therefore an increased risk of type 2 diabetes are not yet fully understood. However, it occurs when people become overweight and exercise less.

A vicious circle can be set up, particularly if there is exposure to a diet high in high glycaemic index foods. Insulin sensitivity decreases and more and more insulin is needed to deal with blood sugars. Blood sugar levels, in turn, rise and more body fat is laid down, thus increasing obesity. This is aggravated by the fact that there is less call on this growing energy base of fat to be broken down in people who exercise less.

Eventually the resistance to insulin is so great that the body is simply unable to produce enough insulin to keep sugar levels under control. Medication is needed to artificially increase insulin levels to try to ward off the complex chronic ill effects of diabetes.

There are a number of factors which can positively influence insulin sensitivity, including the amount of exercise we take and the foods we eat. Both low glycaemic index foods and foods which are high in fibre have a positive effect and so does the monounsaturated oleic acid in olive oil. There have been a number of studies to this effect. A study undertaken by researchers in Rome, and published in 2015 in the journal *Nutrition and Diabetes*, found that there are lower levels of circulating blood glucose and insulin after a meal that includes olive oil. Another from the University of Cordoba, published in *Diabetes Care*, showed that when compared with a high glycaemic index carbohydrate or high saturated fat diet, a diet rich in monounsaturated fat improved blood sugar levels before and after eating. It was also found that the olive oil diet prevented the transport of body fat to the waistline.

Extra Virgin Olive Oil and Diabetes

The effects of olive oil on insulin sensitivity, sugar regulation and the feeling of satisfaction after a meal combine to make it an integral part of the best lifestyle to prevent and also to treat diabetes.

The majority of cases of type 2 diabetes are related to obesity, lifestyle and poor diet. Studies have shown that olive oil has a role in not only reducing the risk of developing type 2 diabetes, but also in lessening the chances of people who are borderline diabetic progressing to full-blown diabetes.

Research from the large Predimed study published in the journal *Diabetes Care* in 2011 demonstrated that the risk of developing type 2 diabetes was reduced by 50 per cent in those on a Mediterranean style diet with olive oil compared with those on a low-fat diet. A different study, The SUN (Seguimiento Universidad de Navarra) study of 13,000 university graduates in Spain showed a reduction in risk of developing type 2 diabetes of 83 per cent in those who adhered to a Mediterranean pattern of eating. Olive oil, as part of the Mediterranean Diet, will also reduce the severity of diabetes in those with established disease, and has been shown to reduce the risk of consequent heart disease and stroke.

With rapidly rising numbers of people in the Western world not only becoming more and more obese but also developing diabetes, with its associated increased risk of heart disease and stroke as well as kidney and eye conditions, the evidence of the protective role of the Mediterranean Diet enriched with olive oil must be integral to any prevention strategy.

Extra Virgin Olive Oil and Thermogenesis

It is necessary for all warm-blooded animals to maintain a body temperature that provides the stability that is necessary for all our systems and organs to work efficiently. The process of producing heat within our bodies is called thermogenesis. We generate heat in three different ways: firstly through exercise-associated thermogenesis (EAT), which is the burning of calories during exercise; secondly through non-exercise activity thermogenesis (NEAT), which is the generation of heat from the ongoing chemical activity in the body; and thirdly, through diet-induced thermogenesis (DIT), which is the processing of the food that we eat.

All of these involve using up energy through the breakdown of fats in storage cells and so may contribute to a reduction in body fat. There is some evidence that after an olive oil-rich meal, there is an increase in thermogenesis, and thermogenesis is one of the ways in which energy is used up, as opposed to being laid down as fat.

The Ultimate Diet?

At any one time, many millions of people in Europe and the USA are adhering to some kind of weight-reducing diet. The trend appears to be that people are engaging in a broader range of different diets for shorter periods of time.

Specific diets come and go. They become fashionable, often because they are promoted by celebrities, and then they fade away as other newer diets come along. They are frequently based on a piecemeal approach rather than on a holistic view of our patterns of eating and lifestyle habits.

However, history has taught us to be sceptical of diets which ignore the complexities of the ways in which our foods and lifestyle interact. We have spent decades replacing fats with sugars, attempting to slash calories or looking for miraculous powders to replace our natural foods. The diet industry is said to be currently worth an astonishing $20 billion per year in the USA alone, but the stark evidence is that most of these diets fail to produce long-term positive results.

Most people diet for the purposes of losing weight rather than for more general health benefits. This is very evident if you look at the numerous commercial diets which are advocated at any one time, many of which are potentially harmful in the combination of weight-loss foods they advise. People who diet in order to lose weight will, of course, gain some benefits if they are significantly overweight in the first place. However, the ultimate diet is one which achieves long-term healthy weight and protects from chronic disease through the consumption of a variety of natural ingredients.

When science scrutinises diets for sustained healthy weight loss and for the broader benefits of reducing the risks of the common chronic diseases to which we are susceptible, there is only one way of eating in the West which offers evidence that is established and compelling and that is a Mediterranean Diet with olive oil at its heart.

In 2012, a study published in the *New England Journal of Medicine* showed that a Mediterranean-style diet with some limits on overall calorie intake but which included 30–45ml of olive oil a day showed successful and sustained weight loss over six years for people who were overweight at the start of the study. It was superior to both a low-fat diet and a low-carbohydrate diet and it provided better cholesterol profiles when the three diets were compared. Participants were also far more likely to stick to the Mediterranean Diet because it was so much more enjoyable!

Summary

1 Olive oil contains the same number of calories as other fats but there is no evidence that regular consumption causes weight gain as part of a healthy lifestyle.

2 The monounsaturated oleic fat in olive oil contributes much less to body fat than other types of fatty foods, such as saturated fats.

3 Glucose derived from refined grains and sugars is more likely to contribute to weight gain than olive oil. This is because these foods have a high glycaemic index.

4 High glycaemic index foods are easily broken down to glucose in the body and so raise blood sugar levels very quickly. Low glycaemic foods, such as whole grains, break down much more slowly and so do not push up blood sugar levels to the same degree.

5 A Mediterranean Diet with olive oil has been shown to promote a healthy weight as well as reducing the risk of a whole range of other chronic diseases.

6 Insulin is the hormone released by the body to regulate the level of blood sugar. Most healthy people only need relatively small amounts of insulin to regulate their blood-sugar levels.

7 Bad diet and obesity can lead to the body needing more insulin to cope with high blood-sugar levels. This can create a vicious circle which can lead to type 2 diabetes and related conditions.

8 Olive oil, low-GI foods and foods which are high in fibre all have a positive effect on this condition.

9 Various studies show that following a Mediterranean Diet which is high in olive oil produces a very marked reduction in the likelihood of developing type 2 diabetes.

10 Millions of people embark on diets of various kinds every year but few of them achieve the desired objective of a healthy and sustained weight loss.

11 With olive oil being an important factor in the prevention of obesity and resultant diabetes as well as in preventing a whole range of other chronic diseases, it seems logical that a Mediterranean Diet with high levels of olive oil should be the universal diet of choice.

OLIVE OIL AT THE HEART OF THE MEDITERRANEAN DIET

THANKS to extensive and ongoing research in many countries we are now able to celebrate the health-giving qualities of extra virgin olive oil. Science has shown that a couple of tablespoons of this excellent fruit juice each day can provide us with unique and powerful health benefits.

Yet olive oil is not a medicine. It is a natural and nutritious food and it is the foundation of the Mediterranean Diet. Olive oil is deeply embedded in the cuisines of the Mediterranean region. It is used to cook, flavour and enhance many traditional dishes which, when analysed scientifically, are shown to have really positive effects on our health. Olive oil not only acts as a first-class cooking medium and flavouring agent, it also brings out the best nutritional qualities of the other ingredients.

Indices used by scientists to score and measure people's adherence to the Mediterranean Diet, increasingly begin with questions relating to the use of olive oil. It is the main source of fat and the foundation of the overall diet, which is rich in vegetables, fruit, fish, nuts and herbs.

The Mediterranean Diet

The phrase 'Mediterranean Diet' was first used by Professor Ancel Keys of Minnesota University who, in the late 1950s and 1960s used it to describe the pattern of eating and lifestyle common to the Mediterranean countries featured in the Seven Countries Study. He found that people who followed this way of eating enjoyed better health and lived longer than people in the affluent countries of north-western Europe and the USA. The phrase subsequently came to be a used as a shorthand for the traditional diet of southern Italy, Greece and Crete.

Today the name describes much more than a single regional pattern of eating. The culinary culture, the cooking techniques and the fresh local produce of the countries around the Mediterranean basin are extremely varied but they all have one thing in common. They all use olive oil every day, often 20–30ml per person per day and perhaps as much as 70ml. In addition, the olive oil is served with fresh, unprocessed ingredients and low levels of meat, simple carbohydrates and refined sugars.

The basis of the diet is fresh, seasonal fruit and vegetables with unrefined, wholegrain cereals, dried pulses such as beans and lentils, nuts and seeds. Fish or shellfish is eaten at least twice a week. Some dairy produce, usually in the form of cheese and yogurt from the milk of grazing sheep or goats, is also regularly included.

Red meat is eaten less frequently and in smaller amounts than is usual in the more affluent diets of northern Europe and the USA. Poultry and game are the more likely choices. Herbs and spices rather than salt are used to flavour and garnish dishes and so add to the nutritional profile of the diet. Dessert usually consists of seasonal fruits, though for special occasions sweets are prepared using seeds, nuts, olive oil-based filo pastry and honey for sweetening. Baked products high in sugar and trans-fats are rare. Wine is often drunk in moderation with a meal and herbal teas are consumed afterwards. The culture of taking time to enjoy the food is central to the lifestyle.

This traditional Mediterranean Diet contains a healthy ratio of fats. It is high in monounsaturated fats, from olive oil, compared to saturated fats from animal sources. The saturated fats that are consumed in the diet tend to be saturated fats such as goat's milk cheese that are not associated with raising potentially harmful cholesterol levels (see page 11). Where red meat is eaten, it is unprocessed and often marinated or cooked in olive oil, wine and herbs, which is thought to reduce harmful compounds that may be produced as a result of frying and grilling. The polyunsaturated fats in the diet have an optimum overall ratio of Omega-6 to Omega-3 polyunsaturated fats of less than 4:1 (see page 14).

The average daily quantity of vegetables eaten is significantly higher in the Mediterranean Diet than in the average modern diet. These vegetables are rich in fibre and in other compounds, such as those which give them their colour. These are called phytonutrients. Olive oil is the medium for cooking and presenting these vegetables dishes and the two together provides a blend of essential vitamins, minerals and antioxidants.

The unrefined wholegrain carbohydrates in the diet are generally low glycaemic index and, particularly when combined with olive oil, have a very low glycaemic load. Pulses and nuts, too, have very low glycaemic load and are excellent sources of vitamins, minerals and fibre.

Olive Oil and the Power of the Mediterranean Diet

The daily inclusion of extra virgin olive oil in the diet contributes to ensuring that the health benefits of the Mediterranean Diet are more than the sum of its parts. It is the most essential element of this pattern of eating. Extra virgin olive oil, in particular, not only complements and enhances the nutrition of the whole diet but also has great benefits of its own in reducing the risks of many chronic illnesses and conditions.

Numerous scientific studies over the years confirm this. The EPIC study (see page 2) has shown that a high intake of olive oil can reduce the risk of death from heart disease by as much as 44 per cent and overall death rates by 26 per cent. The Predimed study (see page 2) also showed that a Mediterranean Diet supplemented with extra virgin olive oil can cut by a third the risk of heart disease, stroke and death in a large population considered to be at risk of cardiovascular disease.

Research is demonstrating that olive oil can be considered protective against disease independent of other dietary elements. In 2016 the journal *Public Health Nutrition* published results from a trial of 1,200 participants in Athens which showed an association between exclusive use of olive oil rather than other cooking or dressing oils with a 37 per cent lower likelihood of developing heart disease even after taking into account other risk factors and lifestyle choices, including physical activity and diet. The authors of the paper concluded that this reduced risk with the use of olive oil was regardless of the population's adherence to the Mediterranean Diet.

Reduced Risk with the Mediterranean Diet

Since Ancel Keys first observed the reduced levels of many chronic diseases in the area of the Mediterranean Diet with olive oil, more research has described the powerful effects of the diet on health.

The Mediterranean Diet with olive oil is associated with a reduced risk of:

- heart disease and mortality from heart disease

- strokes

- high blood pressure

- high cholesterol

- dementia, including Alzheimer's Disease

- many forms of cancer

- Parkinson's Disease

- kidney disease

- developing type 2 diabetes

- erectile dysfunction

- arthritis

- osteoporosis

- asthma

- depression

- inflammatory bowel disease

- premature death

Ageing and DNA

The Mediterranean Diet achieved headlines recently for 'slowing the process of ageing'. This related to a study which looked at the DNA in human cells – the most fundamental central programming of our bodies.

Strands of DNA, which makes up our chromosomes, have protective caps called telomeres. These caps gets shorter every time a cell divides, and are subject to further shortening from inflammation and oxidative stress. Shorter telomeres are considered to be markers of ageing, with longer telomeres associated with longevity. As part of a long term Nurses Health Study looking at over 4,000 women it was found that closer adherence to a Mediterranean Diet was linked to the presence of longer telomeres. So, the Mediterranean Diet seems to protect our DNA from some of the processes of ageing.

A Healthy and Long Life

Reducing the risk of illness means that there is an increased likelihood of enjoying a full, healthy and longer life. There are, of course, some factors, such as our genetic make-up, which cannot be altered. However, it is possible to choose a lifestyle and pattern of eating which is enjoyable and which can also maximise the possibility of remaining fit and well into old age.

In one of a series of studies undertaken by researchers at the University of Palermo in Sicily, healthy 90-year-olds showed that they were most likely to have remained faithful to the traditional Mediterranean Diet.

Further evidence has shown even more powerful effects of the Mediterranean Diet, particularly when part of a broader healthy life-style. One study in 2011 from Maastricht University in the Netherlands, published in the *American Journal of Clinical Nutrition* suggested that a population of non-smoking women of a healthy weight who adopted a Mediterranean Diet along with regular exercise might enjoy 15 more years of life by adopting such ways of living. The equivalent estimate for men was eight years.

Researchers studying the Spanish subset of the EPIC study even quantified the reduction in risk of developing heart disease, observing a 14 per cent lower risk for each tablespoon of extra virgin olive oil consumed per day. This was double the effect when compared with olive oil that was not described as extra virgin. The increase in protection with increasing quantities of extra virgin olive oil has been described in studies which have generally looked at consumptions of up to 3 tablespoons of the oil.

The decline in mental functioning, and ultimately a diagnosis of dementia, is one of the greatest fears of old age. However, the Predimed study (see page 2) found that those people with no existing problem of mental functioning, who adhered to a Mediterranean Diet supplemented with extra virgin olive oil each week showed consistently better cognition over a four-year period as the study progressed in comparison with those on a standard low-fat diet.

While it may not reverse the condition, there are suggestions that extra virgin olive oil may also be beneficial to those already suffering from dementia. There is some tantalising animal research where genetically susceptible mice were fed oleuropein, an antioxidant in extra virgin olive oil. Although it is difficult to extrapolate to humans, the supplemented group showed far fewer nerve tangles and brain plaques seen in dementia and also performed better in simple tasks which measured memory of cognitive performance.

Other changes in the brain which are seen in older people who have a decline in memory and performance is that of brain shrinkage, or atrophy. A study published in the journal *Neurology* looking at populations with an average age of 80 years in Manhattan showed an association between a high Mediterranean Diet score and a larger brain size. Headlines in the news suggested that the diet slows the ageing process by five years!

Feel-good Factor

It has been shown on numerous occasions in different settings that what we eat can have a profound effect on the way we feel about ourselves and our lives. For example, the SUN (Seguimiento University of Navarra) study looked at the effect of a Mediterranean Diet on the quality of life of a group of graduates in Spain. Participants reported not only better physical health but also better emotional well-being and vitality. A Mediterranean Diet with ubiquitous olive oil can not only prevent diseases but can also have a significant feel-good factor.

Summary

1 The phrase 'Mediterranean Diet' nowadays refers to the traditional ways of eating in the countries surrounding the Mediterranean Sea where the use of olive oil is a fundamental part of the diet.

2 The Mediterranean Diet is synonymous with the regular use of olive oil. Levels of olive oil consumed in these region vary from 30ml to 70ml per person per day.

3 The Mediterranean Diet is made up mainly of fruit and vegetables with unrefined cereals, dried pulses and nuts and seeds with some fish, poultry and dairy products from grazing sheep and goats. Herbs and spices are used for flavouring.

4 The diet contains good ratios of different fats with high levels of monounsaturated fats and an Omega-6:Omega-3 ratio of less than 4:1.

5 Numerous studies attest to the health benefits of this kind of diet, cutting the risks of many chronic diseases by quite substantial percentages.

6 Many of these benefits may largely be due to the olive oil content of the diet. It is very likely that many of these benefits would be lost without the daily use of olive oil.

7 It is impossible to consider the Mediterranean Diet without the unique and powerful inclusion of olive oil. We are beginning to understand the significant contribution made by olive oil to the health we associate with the oil itself and the diet as a whole.

NO COMPARISON! OLIVE OIL AND OTHER OILS AND FATS

UNTIL the mid-twentieth century there were very few vegetable oils other than olive oil. In the West the choice was between olive oil and butter or other animal fats and this choice was largely dictated by region. In those areas around the Mediterranean where olive trees flourished, olive oil dominated. Further north, animal fats were widely used and that preference was taken to the New World of the Americas and beyond.

In the second half of the twentieth century, concerns about the possible harmful effects of eating saturated animal fats led to new advice and people were encouraged to replace butter with polyunsaturated fat. This has resulted in the manufacture of a wide range of different vegetable oils.

Olive oil is still the dominant source of fat in the Mediterranean region but even there many people have moved away from the traditional diet to a diet including the newer vegetable oils processed from sources other than olive oil. Obesity is on the increase in these regions. Greece, in particular, now has a rapidly accelerating problem of weight gain.

The Fats in Vegetable Oils

Vegetable oils were originally named as such to distinguish them from hard fats of animal origin. These oils actually come from seeds, nuts and fruits and they contain varying proportions of saturated, polyunsaturated and monounsaturated fats. Both the total quantity of particular fatty acids and their combinations will have an effect on health.

Predominant Types of Fatty Acids in Oils and Fats

Polyunsaturated fats are found in:	Sunflower seed oil
	Safflower oil
	Soya bean oil
	Corn oil
	Cotton seed oil
Monounsaturated fats are found in:	Olive oil
	Rapeseed oil
	Peanut oil
Saturated fats are found in:	Coconut oil
	Palm oil
	Butter
	Suet

Most vegetable oils, including olive pomace oil, are extracted in high-temperature processes using solvents such as hexane. The process results in relatively cheap oils which are not particularly healthy. The naturally occurring healthy compounds in plants, including the rather low levels of polyphenols, are completely lost. The refining process used for ordinary olive oil does not involve the use of chemicals though the process does remove some, though by no means all, of the health benefits of olive oil.

Extra virgin and virgin olive oils, on the other hand, are extracted without the use of heat or any kind of chemical solvents and so the naturally high levels of polyphenols and antioxidants are not affected. There are also a small number of other vegetable oils which are extracted at relatively low temperatures (40–60°C as compared to 27°C for cold pressed and cold extracted olive oil) without the use of chemicals. Two of these, avocado oil and rapeseed oil, have high levels of monounsaturates. Like extra virgin olive oil, these oils have a long shelf life. They are also resistant to heat during cooking (see page 102).

Cold pressed oils processed from seeds with a high level of polyunsaturated fatty acids, such as hemp oil, are less heat-stable and will break down more quickly than those rich in monounsaturated and saturated fatty acids. They will not stand up to use in cooking and have a much shorter shelf life.

Arguments abound about the health benefits of different vegetable oils, with producers making myriad claims and counter-claims about the virtues of their oils in comparison to other oils. The chemistry to back these up can get quite complex.

The level of absorption of different fatty acids into the body varies depending on the exact form of the triglyceride in which it is carried. Fatty acids may be carried in the first, second or third position of the triglyceride (see page 9). Those which are carried in the second position seem to be well absorbed with lesser amounts being absorbed from the other positions.

In some countries, rapeseed oil has been marketed with the claim that it contains half the saturated fat content of olive oil. In fact, the difference is relatively small. Olive oil contains around 12 per cent saturated fat but it is not very well absorbed as only very small quantities of it are carried at position two on the triglyceride molecule. On the other hand, 50 per cent of the beneficial oleic acid in olive oil is carried at position two and so is very readily absorbed.

A review by Dr Richard Hoffman published in the *British Journal of Nutrition* in 2014 concluded that extra virgin olive oil is healthier than rapeseed oil, giving more protection against disease, and reporting that although rapeseed oil is rich in good fats there is very limited evidence that this translates into any real reduction in disease risk. By contrast, evidence for the health benefits of extra virgin olive oil is very strong and may be linked to the high levels of antioxidants in the oil, which are lacking in rapeseed oil.

Palm oil is one of the few highly saturated vegetable oils and is semi-solid at room temperature. The principle saturated fatty acid here is palmitic acid. Palm oil is widely used in the processed food industry and is now being used in a new 'esterification' process which is taking over from hydrogenation in producing more hardened fats. This chemical process results in a redistribution of fatty acids from their original positions on the triglyceride with a higher proportion of saturated fatty acids being carried in position two. There is some concern that these new processed fats will have the same potential to cause harm as the trans-fats formed by the hydrogenation process.

Coconut oil is also rich in saturated fat, containing even more than butter. The saturated fat in unrefined coconut oil is a medium-chain saturated fat which is considered by some to be less likely to raise potentially harmful LDL cholesterol. However, when coconut oil is refined, the use of high temperatures and solvents means that it loses some of its nutrients and it may even be partially hydrogenated.

Cotton seed oil is widely used in America where it is a popular kitchen oil. It is predominantly made up of polyunsaturated fatty acids of which Omega-3 linolenic acid accounts for 18 per cent. This can be something of a problem as linolenic acid is particularly unstable. There are also relatively high levels of saturated fat but this is in the form of lauric acid which is a medium-chain saturated fatty acid and so not considered to be as harmful as long-chain fatty acids.

The Saturated Fat Debate

Until very recently, saturated fat was cast as the villain of the piece but there are now important changes in our understanding of the effect of saturated fats. There is indeed a link between high consumption of saturated fat and rising levels of LDL or 'bad' cholesterol. This is particularly true of those saturated fats that are found in some dairy and meat products. There is also an association between high levels of LDL and heart disease.

However, there is still a good deal of debate about exactly how these links work. There seems to be contradictory evidence about whether there actually is an increased risk of dying from raised levels of saturated fat in the diet. The predicted rise in mortality does not appear to have been proven beyond doubt. Some academics question the validity of drawing conclusions from a combined analysis of a large number of different studies. They believe that the differences in the details of the many studies make it impossible to extrapolate this kind of conclusion.

Others argue that the reason that there has been no change is that saturated fats have been replaced in our diet with other potentially harmful substitutes, such as high Omega-6 polyunsaturated fats and sugars.

Studies also generally fail to take into account the different types of saturated fat, some of which are more likely to raise cholesterol than others. Nor do they include the fact that, depending on their structure and their place on the triglyceride molecule, some saturated fats are absorbed much more easily than others.

The Minor Constituents of Oils That Are Not so Minor

Fats make up between 97 and 99 per cent of extra virgin olive oil, however it is the 1 to 2 per cent of so called 'minor constituents' which perhaps have the greatest effect on health. These include hydrocarbons, tocopherols, phenolics, sterols, chlorophyll, carotenoids, terpenic acids and other volatile compounds which in particular contribute to the taste and aroma of olive oil.

Many of these chemicals have antioxidant effects, protecting the oil from deterioration, but more significantly they are also the most important factors in the health benefits of olive oil, perhaps in the health benefits of the Mediterranean Diet as a whole.

There is a big difference between the oil derived from a fruit and that from a seed. Fruit is exposed during slow ripening to potentially harmful external stresses from heat, light and the atmosphere. Fruit trees have evolved to produce a complex array of compounds, including antioxidants, which are protective of the developing seeds as they mature and until the fruit is ready for dispersal. The oils produced from fruits such as olives and avocados tend to be very much higher in these complex compounds than oils from seeds.

Summary

1 There is now a wide range of vegetable oils on sale. Some are rich in polyunsaturated fatty acids, others are rich in monounsaturated fatty acids and some are predominantly saturated.

2 Oils with high levels of polyunsaturated fatty acids are not as stable as those which are high in monounsaturated fatty acids, such as olive oil.

3 Palm and cotton seed oils have quite high levels of saturated fatty acids in their make-up and are not so healthy. Coconut oil, too, is rich in saturated fat but here the saturated fats are medium-chain rather than long-chain fatty acids.

4 The level of absorption of fatty acids into the body depends on the exact position they occupy on the triglycerides on which they are carried. In olive oil, 50 per cent of the oleic acid is carried at the most advantageous position with only 10 per cent of the saturated fat carried in this position.

5 Ratios of Omega-6 to Omega-3 in the modern Western diet are very high and increasing the consumption of olive oil helps to reduce this ratio. This is not because olive oil has very much Omega-3 itself but because substituting Omega-9 for Omega-6 reduces the Omega-6:Omega-3 ratio in the diet as a whole.

6 The non-fatty acid components of olive oil are those which contribute most to health and they are not present in most other vegetable oils.

PART 2

CHOOSING AND
USING OLIVE OIL

OLIVE oil is produced in all the countries surrounding the Mediterranean Sea and increasingly elsewhere in the world in regions that enjoy a Mediterranean climate. Within these main areas there are often many different regions producing olive oil and each of these has their own indigenous olive varieties and methods of cultivation, production and extraction. The result is a huge range of different oils with different flavours and different health benefits.

This potentially enormous choice has become increasingly available around the world as non-producing countries import and gradually use more olive oil. Olive oil is now on sale in a wide range of shops in many countries. More is on sale via the internet. However, not all these oils are the same and choosing the right oil is very important.

MAKING THE GRADE – NOT ALL OLIVE OIL IS THE SAME

Olive oil is the freshly pressed juice of the olive fruit with the water removed. Under the mandatory regulations set up by the International Olive Council (IOC) and the European Union, olive oil must be obtained from the fresh fruit of the olive only by mechanical or other physical means under conditions which do not lead to degradation of the oil. All olive oil comes from a single or first press. This has been the case since the introduction of the hydraulic press at the end of the nineteenth century.

The resulting oil must come up to the standards required for virgin or extra virgin status for it to be bottled and sold as such. If it does not come up to these standards it is sent to a refinery where it is cleaned up and then flavoured with a little virgin or extra virgin oil and sold simply as olive oil. No chemical solvents are used in this process.

The residue of stones and flesh which remains after the extraction of the oil is known as pomace. It still contains a small quantity of oil. This oil is extracted with the use of solvents and then refined, the total process stripping the oil of all its non-fatty acid components. Like ordinary olive oil, it is mixed with a little virgin or extra virgin olive oil to sell as olive pomace oil.

Fresh Is Best

Olive oil is best when it is fresh. Once the olive has been picked the oil in it starts, very gradually, to deteriorate. There are numerous factors during harvesting and processing which can speed up this deterioration to the point where the oil is not fit for human consumption. Transport and storage conditions can also affect the quality of the oil. In addition, there is a possibility of adulteration with other cheaper oils. All of these issues mean that only about half of the oil produced in the world needs no further processing.

Originally the only way to judge an oil was by tasting it. This was often done by a single person and was very subjective. Today, chemical tests have been developed to set the standards for extra virgin status. These tests are carried out in special laboratories which are accredited by the IOC.

However, taste still plays a very important role in the judgement of extra virgin olive oils. It has been shown that the human nose can detect the defect of rancidity at concentrations as low as 1:10,000 dilution. This is a level at which normal chemical testing might not be able to show a measureable difference. Specially trained tasting panels have been set up to recognise faults such as rancidity and others. Rigorous guidelines are laid down for the methodology and procedures used by the panels and the panels themselves are regularly checked. The result is that the subjectivity of tasting has almost completely been eliminated. The results of a panel in Spain, for example, will be within a very small percentage point of the results from a panel in California or Italy.

Grades of Olive Oil

Here are the main grades which you are likely to find in the shops in descending order of quality. Each grade has an official description which must appear on the label of the bottle; these descriptions are given in italic.

Extra Virgin Olive Oil

'Superior category olive oil obtained directly from olives and solely by mechanical means.'

This is the top grade of olive oil. It is the natural juice of the olive with the olive water removed. Its free acidity level must not exceed 0.8g per 100g. It must also have fault-free aroma and flavour.

Virgin Olive Oil

'Olive oil obtained directly from olives and solely by mechanical means.'

This is the next grade of olive oil. It, too, is the natural juice of the olive with the olive water removed. Its free acidity level must not exceed 2g per 100g. It must also have fault-free aroma and flavour. Very little of this category is sold in the shops. It is used mainly in food production.

Olive Oil

'Oil comprising exclusively olive oils that have undergone refining and oils obtained directly from olives.'

This oil is obtained by blending refined olive oil and virgin or extra virgin olive oil. Its free acidity level must not exceed 1g per 100g. In some countries this is known as 'pure' olive oil. There are no rules regarding the percentage of virgin oil that is added back and this can vary from very little to as much as 50 per cent.

Olive Pomace Oil

'Oil comprising exclusively oils obtained by treating the product obtained after the extraction of olive oil and oils obtained directly from olives.' Or 'Oil comprising exclusively oils obtained by processing olive pomace oil and oils obtained directly from olives.'

This oil is obtained by extracting and refining oil from the pomace residue left after the extraction of olive oil and blending with virgin or extra virgin olive oil. Its free fatty acid level must not exceed 1g per 100g.

Acidity Levels in Olive Oil

Acidity levels are set for each grade of olive oil with 0.8 per cent as the maximum for extra virgin status. However, good-quality extra virgin oils will often have acidity levels of 0.4 per cent or even lower.

The acidity test measures the free fatty acid content of the oil. There are a number of different fats in olive oil which are commonly bound together in groups of three. So-called free fatty acids are released when these groups start to break up. This can happen as a result of diseased fruit, delays between harvesting and extraction of the oil, careless extraction processes resulting in damaged or bruised fruit, excessive temperatures at pressing and bad storage of the oil.

The free fatty acid or acidity level not only gives an indication of how the olives and the oil have been treated during harvesting and processing but also of the possible health benefits of the oil. The conditions which lead to high acidity levels also reduce levels of beneficial phenols, antioxidants and vitamins.

Peroxide Test

Oxygen is highly reactive and can cause changes to the chemistry of our foods when they are left exposed to the air. These in turn can cause changes within our bodies, damaging delicate structures and disrupting subtle processes within cells.

Oxidation of olive oil occurs when oxygen in the environment reacts with the fats in the oil, causing breakdown of the chemical structure and the generation of molecules called peroxides. The peroxide test measures the levels of these molecules in the oil. If present in significant quantities, they can be detected by tasting the oil as it degrades and becomes rancid. Peroxide levels are a marker for the state of oxidation of an olive oil. The peroxide value of a good-quality extra virgin olive oil should be less than 20.

The antioxidants naturally present in good-quality olive oil protect, to some extent, against the effects of excessive exposure to oxygen. But if the antioxidants in the olive oil have also been diminished by the process of oxidation they will not be available to confer the health benefits now so widely recognised.

Other Laboratory Tests

Other tests, such as measuring the absorption of UV light at specific wavelengths using a machine called a spectrophotometer, can be even more sensitive in detecting levels of oxidation. A spectophotometer can also be used to detect oils that have been incorrectly or fraudulently classified as superior grade oils, such as extra virgin, when they are not.

Another test to support the authenticity of the grade of an oil is the PPP test. This measures the level of pyropheophytin in an oil. This substance is a natural breakdown product from the green chlorophyll pigment of olives and is present in significant quantities where chlorophyll decomposition has occurred following prolonged storage or heating during refining.

Extra Virgin Status and Rapeseed Oil

Some unrefined rapeseed oils carry the description 'cold pressed' or even 'extra virgin'. In the case of olive oil there are very precise definitions of what these phrases mean. However, there is no meaningful definition of what they mean for rapeseed oil. Most producers' literature states that the oils are pressed at 'temperatures below 40°C' which is a good deal higher than the 27°C required to label olive oil as cold pressed or cold extracted and they are not tested for acidity or oxidation.

Importance of Classification

The classification of an olive oil is important because it gives an indication of the quality of an oil and what has happened to it during extraction. The broad categories that are used to describe olive oil do not note the nutritional qualities of the oil, such as phenols or vitamins, but they do illustrate the key characteristics which begin to predict the most healthy oils.

Oil which is simply labelled 'olive oil' has been refined to remove all impurities. This process also removes almost all of the non-fatty acid components which are the source of many of the healthy properties of olive oil. However, refining does not change the monounsaturated fatty acid profile of the oil and around 35–40 per cent of the vitamin E content also remains. So these oils still have more health benefits than other vegetable oils (see page 56).

Refined olive oil is mixed with a quantity of virgin olive oil to give it some flavour. Depending on the quantities added there will also be slightly greater health benefits. Quantities of added virgin oil vary from region to region depending on the perceived preferences of the market. In Greece, for example, where olive oil is really appreciated, quantities of added virgin oil can be as high as 40–50 per cent. Compare this to the 11–12 per cent of Western Europe or the 4–5 per cent of so-called 'light' olive oils. The latter description is often incorrectly interpreted as light in calories when actually these oils are light in virgin oil and so light in taste.

Virgin and extra virgin oils retain all their natural components. However, they still vary in their acidity and peroxide levels. There are, of course, other factors which contribute to the levels of beneficial nutrients in olive oil, but there is a considerable overlap with the conditions which cause free fatty acid levels to rise and those which reduce levels of antioxidants. So low levels of acidity and low levels of peroxides in oils denote low levels of free fatty acids and little oxidation, which in turn are markers of high-quality production techniques. In addition, extra virgin oils with low levels of acidity and generally higher levels of phenols will be more resistant to degradation and oxidation during cooking.

More Categories of Regulations

There are some newer certification systems for olive oil which go much further than the standard IOC and EU tests for extra virgin status. These may be compulsory or voluntary systems run by various bodies in the producing regions concerned.

Californian Standards
A voluntary seal of approval from the Californian Olive Oil Council, for which Californian producers could apply, has now become law in that State. The regulations are stricter than the European standards and it is hoped that all olive oil imported into the US will eventually be subject to the same standards. The acidity level is set at 0.5 per cent rather than 0.8 per cent and the peroxide limit is 15 rather than 20. As yet there is no indication that nutritional measures will be included in the regulations.

Australian Standards

New regulations set for olive oil produced in Australia are the same as those for European oil.

High Standard or HS Accreditation

HS is one of the truly independent certification systems. It is organised and run by the Mastri Oleari or Oil Masters Corporation in Italy but the testing is carried out by another independent organisation, and oils from anywhere can be submitted for inclusion. The standards required for HS status are higher than those for extra virgin status, which call for a minimum level of oleic acid of 55 per cent and an acidity level of 0.8 per cent. For HS certification these levels are 70 per cent and 0.5 per cent respectively. HS certification also requires the measurement of the vitamin E content. The oils for HS certification are analysed and checked at every stage of production.

Geographical Categories of Olive Oil

Olive oils from a specific geographical area can apply for Protected Designation of Origin (PDO) status or for Protected Geographical Indication (PGI) status. Depending on the language of the country of origin, these oils will be labelled AOP, DOP or DO.

Oils which have PDO status are guaranteed to come from the designated region and to have been produced from olives grown and pressed in that area under the relevant PDO regulations. However, PDO status does not guarantee quality. In some regions the thresholds for chemical analysis are the same as those for extra virgin status, in others they are more stringent. However, obtaining the full facts for a particular region is not an easy task.

Oils which have the lesser PGI status merely have to be produced within the geographical area and to have a reputation attributable to that area.

Organic Oils

Organic certification guarantees a low level of chemical residues but it does not necessarily guarantee quality. The same factors that affect the antioxidant and phytonutrient content of non-organic oils also apply to organic oils. The very best oils are made by people who are dedicated to producing an excellent product. These people make the decisions on a quality rather than a quantity basis. They do not take short cuts or cheat. They may or may not be interested in organic methods but they do care about the land and its traditions and keep chemical interference to a minimum.

Until very recently there has not been much evidence to suggest that there are demonstrable differences in health benefits from organic produce. However, in 2014 a team of research workers at Newcastle University in the UK looked at evidence from 340 different studies and found that concentrations of antioxidants, such as polyphenols, varied from 18 per cent to 69 per cent higher in organically grown crops than in conventionally grown produce.

Olive Oil and Fraud

As a valuable commodity since ancient times, cases of olive oil fraud go back thousands of years. The Romans were well aware of this possibility and adopted a system where olive oil could be traced back to the distributor and producer.

Today, there are a number of ways that unscrupulous producers or traders can increase profits through misrepresentation of olive oil. Authorities in countries which export or import oils have a responsibility to monitor, inspect and enforce regulations to ensure the consistent quality of olive oil. In the UK, new powers have been adopted to check on the status of olive oil bottled in the UK rather than at source.

There are several means by which extra virgin olive oil can be adulterated. The oil may simply not be olive oil at all. The oil may be labelled extra virgin but have cheaper refined olive oil added to it, or it may have been adulterated with other refined oils such as hazelnut oil which has a similar fat profile to olive oil. The consequences for health can be very serious indeed when oils are contaminated by or mixed with, for example, nut oils.

Even if the fraudulent oil is not harmful, the consumer is buying an inferior product which will not confer the health benefits associated with the extra virgin oils they are expecting. The extent to which fraud is a problem is very difficult to estimate. This is partly because fraud is not always easy to detect and some fraudulent oils taste perfectly all right for the first few months of their life.

The problem is made more difficult by the fact that not all faulty oils found on the shelves are fraudulent. Olive oil naturally deteriorates over time and this process may be accelerated by exposure to heat and to light. Oils which reach the required standards when they are tested after extraction may have deteriorated more quickly than usual because of factors such as bad conditions during storage and transport. For example, bottles are often displayed in sunny windows or under strong lights, which will subject the oil to both heat and light.

In addition, there is also a good deal of pressure from the retail trade to keep prices down and mass-produced extra virgin olive oil may be at the very edge of extra virgin status when it is tested, with acidity and peroxide levels close to the maximum. These oils simply will not have the shelf life of oils with lower readings and may deteriorate before they are sold.

Any of these factors may contribute to the fact that random checks on oils offered for sale in the shops often reveal a number of olive oils which do not come up to the standard required for extra virgin status. However, not all these checks are scientifically based and so may not reflect the full picture of the many olive oils on the shelves. Despite the various problems, the IOC and EU regulations, which have been reinforced, do ensure that the majority of oils on the shelves are what they say they are.

Summary

1 Olive oil is the fresh juice of the olive fruit with the water removed.

2 There are a number of different grades of olive oil. All are obtained from the first and only pressing of the olive fruit.

3 To be labelled 'extra virgin', olive oil must pass a series of chemical tests and be approved by an organoleptical tasting panel.

4 Classification is important as it not only gives an indication of the quality of the oil, but also illustrates the key characteristics which begin to predict healthy oils.

5 In addition to EU and IOC standards, there are a number of other certifications and seals to identify oils of a particularly high quality.

6 Geographical categories of olive oils, such as PDO and PGI, only guarantee the origin of the oil; they do not guarantee quality.

7 There is currently no research to indicate that unfiltered oils are any better than filtered oils. Organic extra virgin olive oils probably contain more polyphenols that those produced by conventional means.

8 Faulty and fraudulent oils do appear in the market place from time to time. Oils which genuinely reach the standards for extra virgin status may deteriorate faster than usual due to bad storage and transport conditions. A few extra virgin oils have been adulterated by the addition of refined olive oil or cold pressed nut oils. However the majority of oils on the shelves are indeed what they say they are.

FROM SUN AND SOIL
TO LIQUID GOLD

OLIVE trees thrive in a Mediterranean type of climate where the summers are hot and dry and the winters are cool. As a result, commercial production of olive oil is concentrated in the countries which surround the Mediterranean Sea. Olive trees have now also been planted further afield in those countries of the northern and southern hemispheres which also have a Mediterranean type of climate. Olive oils from California, Argentina, Chile, Australia, New Zealand and South Africa have come onto the market. Even newer plantings with experimental groves are springing up in parts of India, Nepal, Pakistan, Uzbekistan and China.

However, there is a good deal more to consider when looking at the production of the finest extra virgin olive oils than the overall climate. The planting and nurturing of the trees, the timing of the harvest and the way in which the oil is pressed, stored and bottled all have a very real effect not only on the quality and taste of the oil but also on the characteristics which affect our health.

In the Grove

Everything that happens in the olive grove sets the scene for the growth of healthy trees and first-class fruit, which in turn lead to the best and healthiest olive oils. This, of course, includes the weather so there will inevitably be some variation in overall quality from year to year. Nevertheless, decisions taken by the growers will still have a significant effect on the finished product.

Planting and Cultivation

In the earliest olive groves that still survive, the olive trees grow in a free and unregulated way with an unplanned mixture of local varieties, but today these old groves are few and far between. Instead, the extensive groves of the twentieth century are planted in rows with the trees set at regular intervals. The spaces between the trees and the rows vary according to the theories on best practice prevailing at the time.

Where there is plenty of space and the land is not too craggy, new methods of high-density and super high-density planting are being adopted in an attempt to produce more olives per square hectare. The trees are set very close together and are trained on wires rather like vines, while much wider spaces are left in between the rows to allow for mechanised harvesting.

The trees are irrigated and fertilised from the start and their development to full maturity is much faster than the traditional five to ten years. In addition, weed killers are used to keep the land clear between the rows and more chemicals used to protect the trees from pests.

There are concerns that this type of farming may create a downward spiral with changes to beneficial insect communities and microbial colonies in the soil leading to the need for even more chemicals! On the positive side, there is an increasing interest in understanding the biodiversity of the olive grove and how the existing ecosystem affects the quality of the environment and ultimately the oil produced.

Stress, Irrigation and Fertilisation

An important factor in the level of antioxidants in olive oil is the degree of natural stress experienced by the olive trees. Stress from factors such as excessive heat, drought, poor soil, UV light and pest infestations encourages trees to produce more polyphenolic antioxidants in the fruit.

It is sometimes said that olive trees like stress and that is why olive groves are often found in craggy, upland areas with poor soil and little water. In fact, the reason why they have traditionally been planted in these conditions is that nothing else will grow there and olives will. If you plant olive trees lower down the slopes or even on flat land they grow very well and produce higher yields. However, it is true that the higher the olives are planted and the more challenging the conditions in which they grow the more likely the fruit is to contain high levels of protective antioxidants.

In many areas, irrigation has been introduced into the groves to combat some of the extremes of the Mediterranean climate and to increase yields. But continuous over-irrigation is detrimental to the quality of the oil both in terms of flavour and polyphenol production.

Unfortunately, there is also a strong temptation to further increase yields by so-called 'fertigation'. Here, a computer-controlled irrigation system carries nitrogen fertilisers to feed the trees on a regular basis. But nitrogen fertilisation tends to reduce polyphenol levels. Such systems can help to satisfy demand but could be at the expense of the quality and health benefits of the resulting oil. In addition, the trees in modern intensive groves are all relatively young and polyphenol levels in the fruit are lower in young trees than in older trees.

In the best run groves, irrigation is only used sparingly. Minimal irrigation increases the stress response in the olive trees and so increases the concentration of protective polyphenols. Fertilisation is kept to a minimum. The trees are usually of mixed ages as very old trees are replaced or the groves are extended with new plantings. Quality will be high with plenty of healthy polyphenols.

Organic Methods of Production

In the more traditional groves a degree of vegetation is allowed to grow between the trees. This may be controlled by ploughing in from time to time or by the grazing of sheep or other animals. The land benefits from the natural fertilisation from the cut vegetation or from the animals. Such groves, often rich in bird and insect life, provide a unique and diverse ecosystem in which healthy olives can thrive.

Organic farmers recognise the value of the olive tree as part of a natural ecosystem which is known to work. Most olive groves do not usually need large applications of herbicides or pesticides and organic farmers only use natural fertilisers or the waste from the pressing of the olives. Pest control is only by organically certified methods and farmers welcome the presence of birds and insects, some of which can cause problems but others can be beneficial.

Varieties

There are hundreds of different varieties of olive and at least 30 to 40 of them are produced on a commercial scale. Some are best suited to the production of olive oil and others are grown predominantly for use as table olives. Each variety has its own special characteristics which contribute to the taste and flavour of the oil it produces and to the health benefits it offers.

Some olive varieties have a naturally high concentration of phenols and aromatic compounds, which give the oils made from them not only unique tastes and flavours but also better antioxidant proper-ties. The latter contribute to our health and also to the lasting qualities of the oil. Others contain fewer phytonutrients and, as a result, the oils made from them tend to age faster. Some olives yield very bitter or peppery oils, others are naturally much sweeter (see page 88).

Most producing regions have their own particular varieties of olive, some of which are not grown outside that area. Traditionally the oil in a region was produced from a random mix of these varieties. However, more and more areas are benefiting from research to find which varieties or clones of varieties are best suited to the local soil and climate and large groves are being planted with varieties that are not indigenous to the region. Producers harvest and process the different varieties separately and blend the resultant oils to various specifications.

At the same time, the use of indigenous varieties is being preserved in the Protected Designation of Origin (PDO) regions. The regulations for these areas specify the varieties which qualify for the designation. Enthusiastic local growers are also reviving varieties which were not the commercial choice in the past.

Outside the traditional producing regions there is no pressure to stick to local varieties, if indeed there are any. Groves in Australia, South Africa or New Zealand, for example, may be planted with Greek varieties side by side with Italian and Spanish varieties.

Harvesting

The finest olive oil with the best health qualities is produced by the most careful harvesting and gentle but quick handling from tree to mill. If the olives are soiled, damaged, stored incorrectly or at the wrong temperature or if there is a delay in processing, damaging oxidation will take place. This results in low-quality oil with a poor taste and low levels of antioxidants. The oil may not even reach the standards required for extra virgin status.

The Timing

The decision how and when to harvest is one of the most important choices the farmer makes. It will influence the cost, the yield and also the quality of the oil. Most varieties of olives ripen for a four to six week period during which the colour changes from light green to purple and black. The skin is the first part of the fruit to change colour, followed by the flesh.

The oil content of the olive increases as it ripens from green to purple but the phenolic and aromatic substances which give the oil much of its quality, flavour and nutritional qualities peak while the olive still has some green colour and start to fall off as it ripens further. For the very best oils the optimum point at which to harvest is at this peak; yields may be smaller but quality will be excellent.

There is a clear-cut difference in the chemical composition of an oil which is made from olives picked 20 days either side of the optimum. This difference in composition affects the colour, the flavour and the antioxidant levels of the oil. Oil from olives with a high percentage of unripe fruit among them results in a more aromatic oil with higher levels of polyphenols. Oil from riper fruit tends to be less bitter and peppery and contain a lower level of polyphenols. This is generally true whether the variety naturally produces a delicate oil or a robust oil.

In the past, farmers believed that the riper the olive the more oil it would contain and so they left the olives on the trees until they fell off, resulting in very bad oil. In fact, the oil content in the fruit peaks not very long after the production of the non-fatty acid components stops.

Harvesting Techniques

Olives damage easily and so the way in which they are handled during the harvest is very important. Once damaged, the oil in the flesh starts to oxidise or ferment. Oxidation reduces the level of antioxidants in the oil and the quality of the final oil. Olives are 'hand-picked' with hand-held rakes, sticks or electrical vibrating combs which dislodge the olives onto nets laid beneath the trees. Only a very few groves are literally picked by hand.

Hand-picking is a very labour intensive procedure and costs are rising everywhere. In addition, people are increasingly unwilling to carry out back-breaking work in the groves. As a result, various types of mechanical harvesting machines have been developed to cut the number of people required for the harvest.

There are tree vibrators which embrace the main trunk and vibrate, causing the fall of the olives, and there are branch shakers for use with larger trees. Harvesting of super-density groves is very highly mechanised with straddle harvesters travelling the rows and brushing the olives into hoppers on the side of the machine.

Mechanical harvesting methods help to speed up the harvest and allow more of the olives to be picked within the optimum period. Any damage done to the olive is offset by the speed at which it reaches the olive mill. This in turn is important in the retention of polyphenols and aromatic compounds and so to the quality of the oil.

In warm or hot weather the olives must be milled as soon as possible after harvesting otherwise they will heat up and start to ferment. In general practice, this means within 24 hours. On some estates the mill is situated on site and the olives can be milled within four hours.

In the Mill

Getting the olives to the mill in good condition is only the first stage of the production of olive oil. The many variables in the extraction process can also result in big differences in the composition of the oil and hence its quality, taste and nutritional benefits.

Processing

At the mill, the olives may still be crushed traditionally by means of granite millstones and hydraulic presses, but this is increasingly rare. The method is labour intensive, slow, open to the air and difficult to keep clean. But when it is carried out with care, it can produce excellent oil with good flavour and high levels of polyphenols.

More usually, olives are processed though one of the various generations of continuous centrifugal presses, comprising a crusher, a stirring machine and one or two centrifuges to separate the oil from the waste vegetal matter and water. This is a very efficient way of processing large quantities of olives in a relatively short time.

The most up-to-date equipment is extremely flexible and it is possible to vary both the speed and the temperatures at all stages of the process. It will also give good results regardless of whether the fruit is very wet or very dry. Very little water is required and the process can work under nitrogen to minimise oxidation. The results are fine oils with really high polyphenol contents.

There are also some other systems which are used for the partial extraction of very high-quality oils such as the Sinolea equipment and the Acapulco process. These are essentially free run systems and the paste left from these processes goes through a hydraulic or centrifugal system to extract the rest of the oil. One of the most recent methods of production is the Denocciolato method. Here the olives go into a kind of grating machine which removes the flesh from the stones, which are then discarded. The flesh then passes through a mixer and centrifugal decanter in much the same way as in normal production.

There are various claims about the benefits of the different systems but more research is needed in all areas before any pronouncements can be made on which system is 'the best'.

However, it is true to say that very good-quality oil can be produced by any of these methods and so can very bad oil. After all, it is just as easy to cut corners, ignore good hygiene practice and generally cheat in a modern mill as in an old-fashioned one.

Storage

Once the oil has been produced it is generally stored in large stainless steel containers which may be sealed with protective layer of nitrogen or argon gas, which prevents oxygen contact with the oils (inert gas blanketing). In such large storage facilities, variations in temperature are reduced and the oil keeps well until it is required for bottling and transport to retail outlets.

In the Market Place

As the worldwide demand for olive oil has grown, so production has increased and now both extra virgin and ordinary olive oil are bought and sold on the international commodity market. This means that mass-produced branded oils and supermarket own-label oils are often made up of a blend of olive oils from a number of different countries. They are bottled by large packing companies which do not produce the oil themselves and buy mainly on price. Provided that the oils come up to the standards required for each grade of oil when they are tested, these companies are rarely interested in the taste profiles or health benefits of the oils.

The oil on the international commodity market comes from very large publicly or privately owned olive oil producers or from large co-operatives. It is the choices made by these companies that will determine the quality of the oil that is on the supermarket shelves. There is considerable pressure, from all levels of the market, to keep prices down and competition is fierce. It is not surprising therefore that the temptation to take short cuts and to use cheaper methods of production is strong. Unfortunately such decisions are likely to result in inferior oils. A very small number of companies have gone even

further by passing off refined olive oil as extra virgin olive oil and fraudulently adulterating extra virgin olive oil with unrefined hazelnut oil.

Conversely, some of the larger producers, and particularly some of
the larger co-operatives in Spain and Greece, have trained their many
thousands of members to bring the olives to the mill at the optimum
time before they are fully ripe. They have also led the way in educating
farmers in some of the finer points of best practice in the groves. As a
result, there has been a gradual raising of standards overall, with large
co-operatives producing some award-winning oils. There has also been
an increase in the ratio of extra virgin olive oil to ordinary olive oil
produced in the world.

A smaller section of the olive oil industry is made up of medium-sized
companies with their own olive mills. These companies pack under
brand names or under their own names and they may or may not own
the groves from which the olives come. They are usually in close contact
with the farmers who supply the olives, acting rather like wine negoci-
ants, overseeing cultivation and processing and setting the standards
which should be reached to make premium-quality olive oils.

Finally there are the so-called 'single estate' oils which come from
family-owned farms. This phrase tends to conjure up visions of grand
houses with vineyards and olive groves owned by aristocratic families
such as those found in central Italy and a few parts of Spain and France.
In fact, this type of fine premium oil comes from all kinds of small
farmers with olive groves around the Mediterranean and elsewhere.

The small to medium-sized grower is in a good position to take the
decisions in the grove and at the mill which will lead to the production
of high-quality olive oils with significant health benefits. But as prices
generally fall in the market they, too, are under a great deal of pressure to put maximum production and efficiency before quality. The
philosophy of the growers and their commitment to producing
top-quality oil is the deciding factor in producing the very best extra
virgin olive oil.

Summary

1 Olive trees thrive in a Mediterranean climate and are now grown in many parts of the world which have such a climate.

2 Everything that happens in the olive grove affects the health of the trees, the quality of the fruit and the subsequent oil.

3 Olive trees need a degree of stress to produce good fruit and hence good oil. The high levels of irrigation and fertilisation used in some high-density olive groves result in oils with lower levels of polyphenols than oils from more moderate methods of cultivation.

4 Organic groves usually produce high-quality, healthy oils.

5 The variety of an olive is an important factor in the levels of polyphenols found in oils pressed from them.

6 The timing, methods and speed of harvesting all have an important effect on the healthy qualities of an oil.

7 Careful processing and storage will also help to maintain the quality and health benefits of the resulting oil.

8 The selection of oils on the market varies from blends of oils from large packers who buy oil on the international commodity market through medium-sized producers who both grow and pack oils to small farmers and estates who grow and pack only their own oils.

HOW TO BUY THE
HEALTHIEST OLIVE OILS

THERE is a wonderful variety of olive oils available in supermarkets, delicatessens and online but how do you go about finding those that you like the best and, at the same time, those with the most positive effects on health?

The first step is, of course, to buy extra virgin oil. The grade of an oil really matters. Ordinary olive oil does give you the benefit of its monounsaturated fatty acid content but the refining process removes all of the non-fatty acid components with the exception of a small amount of Vitamin E and it is these that contribute so much to health.

The Connection between Taste and Health Components

The first thing that most people consider when buying an oil is the taste. Is it a robust oil with pungent aromas and peppery flavours or is it more gentle with a soft, fruity taste? Or do the flavour tones lie somewhere in between? Does it have predominantly herbaceous flavour tones or is it full of tropical fruits, tomatoes or nuts?

Personal preferences vary and provided that the oils come up to the standards required for extra virgin status there is no right or wrong. You should buy what you like and you will naturally use more of it. However, the likelihood is that an oil with plenty of bitterness and pepper will have more beneficial polyphenols or other healthy components than a more delicate oil.

The aroma and taste of an oil is dependent on hundreds of chemical compounds, many of which double as antioxidants and anti-inflammatories. For example, the tyrosol group of polyphenols which form the majority of the polyphenol content of olive oils has been shown to relate to the bitter or peppery flavours in some oils. Oleocanthol contributes to the peppery sensation of an oil. Hexanals give some oils their 'green' or 'grassy' tones. Other chemicals are responsible for the aromas of nuts, tomatoes and apples in oil.

However, if your preference is for less peppery olive oils it is undoubtedly better to consume liberal amounts of what may be a lower-antioxidant olive oil than to be discouraged from using any olive oil at all. After all, olive oil is a delicious food not a medicine to be ladled out in measured doses!

Reading the Label

Whether you are choosing an extra virgin olive oil for its flavour or for its health benefits there are certain features which can point to those oils that are most likely to have more bitterness and pepper or to be particularly healthy.

Packing Details and Countries of Origin

There is an increasing recognition of the importance of provenance and traceability in olive oil, as in other foods. Scandals in food production have focused consumers' awareness of the advantages of understanding more about the origins of our food. If you know where an oil comes from it can really help in deciding how good it will be in terms of quality, taste and flavour and in terms of health.

However, finding out the country of origin is not always as easy as it sounds. Many brands and supermarket own-label extra virgin olive oils

The Variety of Olive

The variety of the olive used in any oil has a strong effect, particularly on the flavour of an oil pressed from it but also on the presence or otherwise of healthy polyphenols. Here is a round-up of the olive varieties most commonly pressed for oils.

Variety	Flavour tones	Pungency	Polyphenol levels	Regions
Coratina	Herbaceous	Strong	High	Southern Italy
Moraiolo	Herbaceous	Strong	High	Central Italy
Picual	Fruits	Strong	High	Southern Spain
Cornicabra	Herbaceous/ fruits	Medium	High	Central Spain
Koroneiki	Herbaceous	Medium	High	Greece
Frantoio	Herbaceous/ nutty	Medium/ Strong	Medium	Central Italy
Hojiblanca	Tropical fruits	Medium	Medium	Southern Spain
Leccino	Herbaceous/ nutty	Medium	Medium	Central Italy
Arbequina	Apples and nuts	Delicate	Low	Northern Spain
Picudo	Tropical fruits	Delicate	Low	Southern Spain
Nocellara del Belice	Tomatoes	Delicate/ Medium	Low	Sicily

But it is important to remember that other factors, such as the climate and soils, the timing of the harvest and the growing and processing techniques, will all have an effect on both the taste profile and the polyphenol levels in the final oil.

are made up a blend of oils from a number of different countries. These oils will be labelled as 'produce of the EU'. Alternatively, the label will list the actual countries from which the oils in the blend originate. They are often described as being mild in flavour and research suggests that many of them have relatively low levels of polyphenol antioxidants.

Producers and packers claiming a single country of origin must substantiate that claim or use the phrase 'packed in' rather than 'produced in'. Nor can an oil claim to be the produce of a particular region within a producing country unless it has PDO status. So if you want to know if your oil comes from a single country or is a blend, read the small print carefully.

Extra virgin olive oil which comes from small and medium-sized producers tends to be of a higher quality than mass-produced oils. These producers are proud to put their details on their labels. Some even have tracking systems which enable their customers to trace an oil back to the actual grove that produced the olives for the oil.

Producing Regions and What to Expect

If you know the region from which an oil comes it can be useful in deciding what it might taste like. This information can point to the varieties of olives which might have been used when this is not on the label and to the traditions and practices of the producers.

There are dangers in generalising about typical tastes and flavours but here is a guide to what to expect from the three largest producing countries of the Mediterranean.

Spain

This is the largest producer, supplying half the world's total of two and a half million metric tonnes of olive oil. In some areas, the groves stretch as far as the eye can see. Nearly half the crop comes from Andalucia where Picual, Picudo and Hojiblanca olives thrive. Catalonia, in the north, is another large producing region, with Arbequina as the main variety. Most of the groves in Spain are a long way from the sea and in the summer months it is very hot. In the past the oils tended to be relatively sweet and golden in colour.

However, the introduction of new varieties, modern techniques for cultivation and processing and earlier harvesting have led to a much wider range of tastes and flavours. Styles vary from the lusciously fruity Andalucian oils of Cordoba and Baena with their melon and passion fruit flavours to the sweet and nutty oils of Catalonia in the north. Andalucia also offers lightly grassy oils with fruit and nuts and the distinctively bitter oils of Jaen pressed from the polyphenol-rich Picual.

Most of the olives for these oils are grown by small farmers and processed in the local co-operatives. From here the oil goes to large secondary co-operatives who sell directly onto the market and to the big international packers. The best of the co-operative oils and oils from small to medium-sized growers are bottled on the spot and sold as premium oils under their own labels.

Greece

Around three to four hundred thousand tonnes of olive oil is produced each year in Greece. The polyphenol-rich Koroneiki olive is the main source of Greek olive oil. Kalamata olives are the best known Greek olives but they are rarely used for olive oil. If you see the name Kalamata on a bottle of olive oil it refers to the mountainous region of Kalamata on the western Peleponnese, not to the olive variety. Mani, Laconia and Sparta are also important producing regions.

The olives are grown in small groves and sold either to private mills or to local co-operatives who, in turn, sell the oil on in bulk to large packers. Some oil is sold locally from the mill. Very little Greek oil is bottled by the grower. The pattern is very similar in Crete, the other major producing region in Greece. Olive oil pressed from the Koroneiki olive is consistently herbaceous in character but varies from fresh and grassy to dry and hay-like, depending on the growing conditions. Other varieties are grown in the north of the country and in the islands but most of this oil is consumed at home.

Italy

Thanks to good marketing, Italy is often the first country that comes to mind when talking about olive oil and it is true that olive oil is produced in almost every part of the country and there is a very wide range of taste and flavours. However, Italy actually imports more olive oil than it produces. This is because many of the large olive oil packers are based there. However, Italy does produce a very high percentage of extra virgin olive as against ordinary olive oil.

Each region has its own olive varieties and a host of different micro-climates. Tuscany has become synonymous with the best of Italian oil but within Italy itself only the Tuscans would agree with this proposition. Tuscan olive oils vary in taste and flavour but most are green and pungent with good polyphenol levels. Descriptions of typical flavours include grassy, artichokes, salad leaves and sorrel as well as meadowsweet hay, roasted nuts and chocolate or bitter herbs. A few oils are sweet and fruity, quite lacking the pungency usually associated with this region. Umbria is another important region for premium oils. Here the tastes and flavours are a little softer than those of Tuscany though they are just as varied. Abruzzo and the Molise are also starting to export some interesting green and grassy oils.

However, it is Puglia and Calabria in southern Italy which are the great producing regions. Much of the oil from here is blended with oils from other countries and sold under brand names but some producers are bottling their best extra virgin oils and selling them individually. Styles in the south vary but the oils tend to be quite sweet often with a peppery punch which comes from blending the softer Ogliarolo olive with the more pungent Coratina.

Extra virgin oils from the islands of Sardinia and Sicily are also worth seeking out. Sardinian oils are usually wonderfully herbaceous with fruity fresh flavours and good lasting qualities. Sicily, too, produces leafy oils often with a touch of tomato coulis in their make-up. The oils of Liguria in the north are apple sweet with nuts and a touch of pepper but with only low levels of polyphenols.

Harvest Dates and Best-before Dates

Fresh is best with olive oil. This is because, from the moment it is pressed from the olive fruit, olive oil starts very gradually to deteriorate. As time goes by this process accelerates and the polyphenol antioxidants and other beneficial chemicals start to disappear.

The date of the harvest is the most useful date to know as it shows exactly how old the oil is. Unfortunately, not many labels carry this precise information. However, PDO oils are required to show the date of the harvest and some small producers also choose to give the date.

The 'best before' date is something of a misnomer as far as olive oil is concerned. The general practice is to allow eighteen months after bottling but all oils will have experienced some deterioration in that time and the oils with lower polyphenol levels will have gone rancid. Unfortunately, there seems to be a move in the market place to give two-year best-before dates. In addition, oils from the large packers are often stored for some time before bottling and so could have been around for more than two years.

The large packers say that this is not a problem as the oil is stored under inert gas and so remains fresh. It is true that the loss of antioxidants is relatively small under this kind of storage but there is still some loss due to the work of enzymes in the oil which are not rendered inactive. The exposure to light and air after storage can result in a more rapid decline.

Many retailers will offer discounts on oils from time to time, but avoid those that are discounted because they are probably approaching their best-before date, and they will be unlikely to be at their best.

Phrases on the Labels and What They Mean

'Early harvest' and 'Late harvest': There is a very distinct difference in the style, taste and healthy benefits between oils that are pressed from early picked olives and those which are made from fruit picked later in the season (see page 80). Even an oil which is usually very sweet and delicate will have a greener style, perhaps with some bitterness or pepper, if it is made from early-harvest olives. Oils that are naturally more aggressive will be very bitter and peppery.

Oils labelled 'Late harvest' are now rare. This is something of a culinary loss. Despite their lower levels of polyphenols, these oils did add a wonderful range of nutty, chocolate tastes to the range of flavours that can be found among olive oils.

'Hand picked' and 'Stone milled': These processes may be traditionally appealing and are often undertaken with great care but there is no data to suggest that they are beneficial in terms of the health qualities of an oil.

'First pressed': This phrase appears on numerous labels but it refers to a time long past when the extraction equipment was not very efficient. Half way through the milling process, hot water was added to enable more oil to be extracted. Heat and water have an adverse effect on oil and the second run of oil was not as good as the first. Thus 'first pressed' and 'cold pressed' (see below) oils gained a reputation for being the best. However, at the end of the nineteenth century the hydraulic press was introduced. This press was able to extract more than 90 per cent of the oil at one go and so the description became meaningless.

'Traditionally pressed': The next major change in the production of olive oil was the introduction of centrifugal equipment which crushes the olives and separates out the oil, vegetable water and paste in one continuous process. The phrase 'traditionally pressed' refers to oil which is extracted by the old hydraulic method. In the early days there were claims that the continuous method was more traumatic on the olives and so produced a lower quality, less healthy oil. However, the modern centrifugal system is designed to reduce damage to the olive, to protect against antioxidant loss and to reduce waste.

'Cold pressed' and 'cold extracted': These phrases also hark back to the early days of adding hot water to the paste. Today the phrase 'cold pressed' refers to oil which has been extracted through a traditional hydraulic press at temperatures at or below 27 degrees Celsius. 'Cold extracted' is the phrase which must be used for oil extracted in the continuous system at similar temperatures.

'Special selection' and 'Grand cru': These phrases do not mean anything specific. At best they are simply a marketing strategy to denote an oil which the producer feels is superior to other olive oils.

Health Claims on the Label

It is rare for olive oil labels to carry details of the polyphenol content of the oil, but a few do. The European Food Safety Authority now allows health claims about the effectiveness of some oils with levels of polyphenols which have a measurable impact on protecting LDL cholesterol from the damaging effects of oxidation. To carry a health claim the oils must have a polyphenol content of 250mg/kg or above. In some EU countries the authorities allow producers to express this effect more clearly for consumers as being beneficial for the heart.

Not very many producers have taken advantage of this but as the importance of antioxidant polyphenols becomes more appreciated so such claims are likely to appear.

Practical Considerations

Olive oil is no longer the specialist and elite product that it once was. It is now on sale in supermarkets and general grocers as well as in delicatessens, farm shops and specialist shops. There are also general and specialist retailers online and websites of growers and producers. It is possible to buy a month's supply of olive oil for the price of a good bottle of wine or a subscription to a TV package.

Always try to buy from shops with a good turnover of olive oil and avoid oil which is displayed in the window or under very strong lights. Badly kept oil will oxidise and go rancid, losing its nutritional and health benefits at the same time. Indeed rancid oil is positively bad for you, producing free radicles which are pro-inflammatory.

What Is Available Where?

Supermarkets, general grocers and large online retailers: Most of the oils stocked here will be own label or branded oils with a selection of ordinary and extra virgin oils. The latter tend to be fairly mild in flavour, probably with lower levels of polyphenols and other healthy nutrients. In the larger stores there may also be a small selection of premium olive oils which will be more expensive but which will also have more flavour and be relatively healthier. Information about any of the oils is usually limited.

Delicatessens and farm shops: These stores stock some branded oils but sell mainly premium and single estate extra virgin oils with good flavours and levels of polyphenols. Information on the oils is varied, with some shops offering good shelf labelling and the possibility of tasting.

Specialist shops: The range of oils on sale in these shops is usually more extensive and also more expensive, with premium and single estate oils predominating. Information can be quite good with knowledgeable assistants and the facility to taste the oils before buying.

Growers' and producers' websites: These specialise in online sales of the grower's own oils. They can be interesting because they will stock the full range of oils produced, some of which may not be generally available in the shops. There is usually plenty of information about the varieties used, the harvest dates and the cultivation and extraction techniques. The most sophisticated sites offer tasting notes and recipes.

The Containers

Bottles come in a variety of shapes and sizes and in different colours. Some bottles are green, brown or even blue. Others are made of clear glass. Oils which are packed in dark bottles or cans will be better protected from light, which can cause oxidation. Exposure to strong light can cause a decrease in the antioxidant content of an oil of as much as 40 per cent in six months.

Tin cans are even better at keeping out all kinds of light and keeping the oil fresh. They are the usual choice for larger scale packs of both extra virgin and ordinary olive oil. These large packs tend to be cheaper in price than the same oil packed in bottles but it is a false economy to buy a 10-litre tin if you do not use olive oil in some quantity. It will simply deteriorate before you have consumed it. If you do decide to buy the larger cans check to see that the oil is the same as the one that you are used to having in bottle. Sometimes the quality level is not exactly the same.

Unfortunately you cannot really see one item which might have an effect on the oil and that is the closure. Metal screw-top closures are the best. They are relatively easy to open and they close well to keep out the air. Corks are not as good, as a corkscrew is needed to open them and cork does not exclude the air as well. Bottles which are closed with wax are also messy to open and once the seal is broken may have the same problem of air getting into the bottle.

Some bottles come with a plastic pouring mechanism inserted in the neck; others come with a cork and pourer. These seem to be useful but oil remains in the pouring mechanism and this will oxidise and go rancid much faster than the oil in the bottle.

The Colour of the Oil

A number of producers still pack in clear glass bottles. This is because they believe, backed up by retailers, that people like to see the colour of the oil before they buy it. Customers think that the colour of an oil will tell them something about its style and taste. Oils with a deep green colour, are believed to be grassy in character with an aggressive, peppery style. Golden oils are thought to be sweet and delicate at best, flabby and boring at worst. Those with a kind of khaki colour are thought to fall within the middle of the flavour spectrum.

Unfortunately, the colour of an oil is not a very useful indicator of its style or flavour. Green oils are not always very strong and pungent. It may just be that the particular olive variety naturally gives a very green colour to the oil. Golden oils may well be sweet and delicate but they often also offer a degree of bitterness or pack a very peppery punch and khaki oils may conform to any of the full range of styles, tastes and flavours.

Filtered Versus Unfiltered

Most oils undergo some degree of filtration to remove residual fruit particles and sediment. Some people extol the virtues of unfiltered oils and various claims have been made about possible superiority of taste and nutritional qualities. Whilst unfiltered oils may have a slightly different texture, there is likely to be little difference in the taste of the same oil in its filtered or unfiltered state.

Insufficient research has been published to draw definitive conclusions about any health advantages. The presence of more plant material from the olive might suggest higher levels of polyphenols and other antioxidants but the earlier oxidation of the solid particles is likely to cause earlier loss of nutrients as the oil degenerates more quickly. So, until robust scientific data supports the use of one type over the other, there will remain uncertainty. If you like unfiltered oil use it up even faster than you would other oils.

Infused or Flavoured Olive Oils

For generations, people in the Mediterranean regions have been adding herbs and other ingredients to olive oil to add taste and flavour. Today commercially produced flavoured oils are growing in availability and popularity, particularly among people who do not care for the taste of unflavoured extra virgin olive oil.

Common flavoured oils include those where the oil is combined with herbs such as basil, rosemary and thyme. Citrus fruits may also be added, including lemon, mandarin and even bergamot. Chilli and other spices are also incorporated into a range of infused oils, and there is even a dark chocolate infusion for desserts.

These flavours can be added in various ways. At worst, such oils may have flavour extracts or even artificial flavours added. The better oils are infused with the flavouring ingredient or they may be produced by pressing the olives and fresh herbs or fruits together at the same time. The latter oils are known as 'agrumato' oils in Italy.

It is also important to check the base oil of flavoured oils. Is it extra virgin or is it ordinary olive oil and is it fresh? It is particularly vital to check on truffle oil. The flavour of the truffle is so strong that it can mask rancidity in the oil. Make sure that the oil is freshly infused and has not been on the shelf for too long.

Price as an Indicator of Quality

Prices for extra virgin olive oil can vary from as little as £4 per litre to £20 per litre in supermarkets whilst in delicatessens and specialists outlets prices may reach £30 per litre or more. There have also been exclusive 'concept oils' marketed at prices in excess of £100 per litre!

There is a definite relationship between the quality and the cost of an oil. Low-cost oils tend to be blends of mass-produced oils from the larger packers which simply do not have the range of tastes and flavours of more expensive oils. Nor are they likely to have the same health benefits. It is simply more expensive to produce high-quality premium oils.

However, there comes a point at which price is less indicative of quality. A good deal of the cost of an expensive oil may well be due to elaborate packaging and marketing. If the weather has been favourable and best practice has been followed in the groves and in the mills, the more reasonably priced premium oils are likely to taste as good as more expensive oils and to be just as beneficial.

General Tips for Buying Healthy Oils

- **Choose an extra virgin oil:** Refined oils described just as 'olive oil' have lower levels of many of the compounds beneficial for health.

- **Choose an oil you like and will enjoy regularly:** There's no point in buying a robust oil that will be left on the shelf.

- **Relish the pepperiness:** A little 'kick' in the oil is probably an indication of healthy levels of antioxidants.

- **Enjoy the grassy tones:** Possibly denoting a good level of hexanal compounds.

- **Read the label:** Look to see descriptions of the oil and harvest date, where possible.

- **Get to know the growers:** Provenance may be key to a really good quality and healthy oil.

- **Value your 'liquid gold':** Pay a little more for a really good oil, particularly to use for drizzling and dressing.

- **Think about organic:** For environmental reasons or for the possibility of lower chemical residues and higher antioxidants.

Summary

1 There is plenty of research which links the taste of an extra virgin olive oil to its levels of polyphenols. Any oil which is described as 'robust', 'peppery' or 'bitter' in flavour is likely to be higher in polyphenols than those which are described as 'light' or 'mild'.

2 The variety of olives has a strong effect, particularly on the flavour of an oil pressed from it but also on the presence or otherwise of healthy polyphenols.

3 If you know where an oil comes from it can really help in deciding how good it will be in terms of quality, taste and flavour and in terms of its health benefits.

4 Fresh is best with olive oil. The date of the harvest is the most useful date to know as it shows exactly how old the oil is.

5 Look to see if there are any health claims or polyphenol levels on the label.

6 Always try to buy from shops with a good turnover of olive oil and avoid oil which is displayed in the window or under very strong lights. Choose oil packed in dark-coloured glass bottles or cans.

7 Try to taste the oil before buying rather than make judgements from the colour of the oil.

8 The choice of filtered or unfiltered oil is largely a matter of personal preference.

9 If you are buying flavoured oils check the base oil and the method of production.

LIVING WITH OLIVE OIL

In the traditional producing regions of the Mediterranean, olive oil is an everyday food. It is used for everything from deep-fat frying to baking bread. It is used to lubricate food for roasting, braising, grilling and frying and it also goes into sauces, marinades, dips and dressings. In addition it is used as a condiment to finish and add flavour to dishes like soups, pasta, baked fish and meat casseroles.

Cooking with Olive Oil

Despite the fact that olive oil is the cooking medium of choice for much of the Mediterranean, the most frequently asked question whenever the health properties of olive oil are discussed in the non-producing countries is 'Can I cook with it?' The answer is a resounding YES.

In the past, some people advocated the rather extreme view that extra virgin olive oil should only be used for finishing and dressing dishes and that refined olive oil should be used for cooking. This probably owed more to the saving on the higher cost of extra virgin oil than to any safety or health considerations.

High-temperature Cooking with Olive Oil

In fact, extra virgin olive oil, with its high levels of polyphenolic antioxidants and other beneficial components, is the best choice for virtually all forms of cooking. Indeed, there are many reasons why unrefined extra virgin olive oil is nutritionally much more beneficial to health than refined oils.

In addition to the mass of evidence of the value of extra virgin olive oil at the heart of the Mediterranean Diet, there are other studies that show the nutritional value of cooking particular foods with extra virgin olive oil. For example, the fat-soluble vitamins and other nutrients in vegetables combine during cooking with olive oil, making them much more readily absorbed by the body. This is true of vitamin E from carrots and squashes as well as the healthy lycopene compounds found in tomatoes. The benefit is even greater if the pan juices are served with the fried food.

Fish and shellfish also benefit from frying in extra virgin olive oil as the combination of the two enables higher levels of vitamin E and polyphenols to be absorbed by the body than would be absorbed by eating the fish or the olive oil on their own. In addition, Omega-3 polyunsatured fats in the fish have a relatively low resistance to heat, but this breakdown can be prevented by the antioxidants in olive oil when the two are cooked together.

Not only does olive oil in cooking combine with healthy ingredients from other foods, it can also decrease the production of unhealthy toxins from some other foods.

Deep-fat frying

There is still a good deal of controversy over the question of whether or not extra virgin olive oil should be used for deep-fat frying. The idea that it is not suitable grew from the competition to appeal to consumers by the seed oil producers, who set great store by comparing the temperatures at which oils are described as 'smoking', implying that oils which have a high smoke point will be more resistant to high-temperature cooking and so offer greater benefits.

High temperatures cause the breakdown of complex fat molecules in oils, producing free fatty acids and other molecules which have been changed by reactions with oxygen. These food products have been linked to cancer and heart disease. The production of smoke during high-temperature heating is a sign of such chemical change.

Refined oils tend to have higher smoke points than unrefined oils. For example, smoke points often quoted are around 210°C for refined olive oil and around 220–230°C for other refined vegetable oils. Extra virgin olive oil is usually quoted as having a lower smoke point at around 190°C. Accordingly it was suggested that refined olive oil should be the choice for high temperature cooking and extra virgin olive oil kept for cooler applications.

In fact, the reality is not as straightforward as this. Firstly, unrefined extra virgin olive oils vary in their smoke points. The general figure quoted may be 190°C but this temperature is significantly higher for an extra virgin olive oil that has high levels of antioxidants. The antioxidants protect the oil from the effects of heat and the smoke point can rise to between 210°C and 230°C. This protection extends beyond the first time the oil is used so that a batch of extra virgin olive oil can be used three or four times before it starts to significantly deteriorate.

In addition, any loss of antioxidants towards the end of its life is variable, with many classes of antioxidants, such as lignans and flavones, showing quite remarkable stability even when experimentally heated to 180°C degrees for 36 hours. However, unfiltered extra virgin olive oils should not be used for high-temperature cooking, as the vegetal material remaining in the oil may be susceptible to heat.

The fear of the detrimental chemical breakdown of extra virgin olive oil engendered from certain quarters has not been helped by the fact that most people are not aware of the actual temperatures at which they cook. In reality, most roasting, sautéing and frying at home, even in deep-fat fryer or wok, occurs at temperatures between 140°C and 190°C. The latter temperature is the optimum temperature for deep-frying chips, the highest temperature required to deep-fry any food. All these temperatures are well within the safe parameters for high polyphenol extra virgin olive oils. The problem arises because neither the smoke point of a particular oil nor its polyphenol level is usually given on the label.

Finally, some people worry about whether they should fry food at all if they are thinking about healthy eating. However, a very large study, part of the EPIC Study, published in 2012, which involved surveying more than 40,000 Spaniards about their cooking habits with olive oil, showed no increased the risk of heart disease or other ill-health as result of the liberal use of olive oil in frying. Beneficial effects were also described in a study from Rome, published in the *Journal of Medicinal Food* in 2011, which showed better blood glucose regulation in women with diabetes who were regularly frying food with olive oil. In addition, the recommendations for diet from the European Food Safety Authority (the EFSA) state that 'there is no evidence that olive oil when used for frying is unhealthy'.

Marinating with Olive Oil

When meat is grilled, roasted or fried, it browns and a range of different compounds are produced. Some of these, such as the flavoursome aroma, are desirable but others are not. For example, chemicals known as heterocyclic aromatic amines (HAs) are created during the browning process and these have been shown to be carcinogenic and could be contributing to an increased risk of bowel cancer. Basting with extra virgin olive oil has been found to reduce these harmful HAs. Marinades which contain olive oil and also garlic, onion, red wine and herbs have an even more powerful antioxidant effect, reducing HAs even further.

Poaching with Olive Oil

This is the opposite of high-temperature cooking and extra virgin olive oil makes an excellent base for poaching. It allows the food to cook at a long slow pace, keeping moisture and flavours sealed in. None of the health giving nutrients is lost. The food emerges beautifully moist with

THE OLIVE OIL DIET

tender texture with added flavours from the poaching oil. The oil is also reusable and should not be thrown away after poaching. Leave it to cool, strain and keep for the next batch of cooking.

Baking with Olive Oil

Olive oil is used widely in baking in the countries of the Mediterranean but elsewhere the tradition is to use butter, margarine or other hard fats. However, extra virgin olive oil can be used very successfully to make all kinds of pastries, cakes and biscuits. The methods used can be slightly different but very often they are easier and less time-consuming.

Olive oil-based pastry is particularly easy to make as there is no 'rubbing in' of the hard fat to be done. The dry ingredients are mixed in a bowl and the liquid ingredients in a jug. The liquid ingredients are then poured over the dry mix and stirred in with a fork or wooden spoon. The mixture is then quickly shaped into a ball with the hands, ready to roll out. Olive oil pastry dough tends to have quite a springy texture and so plenty of flour is needed for rolling out and some force with the rolling pin to get a really thin result.

Though it is very easy to make, it is important to follow a recipe for olive oil pastry. Simply substituting a standard liquid measure of olive oil for a gram of butter will result in pastry with a hard rather than a crumbly or flaky texture .

Cakes, too, are easy to make with olive oil and here it is often possible simply to substitute 15ml oil for 25g hard fat. The oil is usually added to the dry ingredients with any other liquid ingredients, such as eggs, milk or fruit purée. There is no need to rub in the fat or cream the mixture. Using olive oil in biscuits produces very short and crispy biscuits but the mixture can be difficult to roll out. The answer is to flatten the ball of biscuit dough with your hands, then to place it between two layers of cling film and to roll it out in this position. Use cutters as normal and a wide knife or palette knife to transfer the biscuits to the baking tray.

Olive Oil as a Flavouring Ingredient

Extra virgin olive oil is not just a cooking medium, it is a flavouring ingredient in its own right. In the producing the countries, a bottle of olive oil is constantly on the move across the dinner table as it is used as a condiment to enhance the food on the plate, even if that food has already been cooked in olive oil. It is drizzled on soups and stews, grilled and roasted meats and fish, pasta dishes and vegetables. In this way any loss of antioxidants during cooking is more than replaced. Extra virgin olive oil is also used in place of butter on bread and rolls, served as a dip to start the meal and added to raw dishes in the form of dressings and salsas.

In cooking, it is also used as a flavouring and here it is important to choose just the right style of oil for each application. Sweet and gentle oils will not swamp the delicate flavours of lamb's lettuce salads, steamed fish or baked chicken and these oils are the best choice for making mayonnaise and for baking cakes. On the other hand oils with more definite characteristics are needed to stand up to the robust flavours of hearty soups, salads with strongly flavoured leaves, pasta dishes and grilled meats.

Specific flavour characteristics, too, are important. The numerous extra virgin olive oils now available offer a range of flavour characteristics from tomato coulis and tropical fruits through artichokes and salad bowl flavours to toasty nuts and even chocolate which can be used to mix and match with different foods to create the best taste sensations.

Looking after Olive Oil

After you have carefully chosen your olive oil and brought it home it needs to be properly looked after. The benefits of extra virgin olive oil lie in its good fats and polyphenol antioxidants and these components can be oxidised by exposure to high temperatures, UV light and air, rendering them less effective in protecting our bodies from the harmful effects of oxidative stress.

To preserve these health benefits at home olive oil should ideally be kept in a dark, cool cupboard away from direct sunlight. However, most cooks like to have their olive oil to hand by the hob. The answer is to buy in manageable quantities, only purchasing large containers if you use a good deal of oil each week and using the oil as soon after buying as possible.

It is not necessary to store olive oil in the fridge. When olive oil cools to temperatures below five to seven degrees (this varies with the composition of the oil) it may become cloudy and form small clumps of white fat. This process is reversed when the oil is warmed again. For many years this was actually cited as evidence of the quality of the oil, but there is no evidence that there is any effect on taste or health properties for better or worse. However, olive oil should not be frozen. Oil which has been frozen tastes fine when it is first thawed but deteriorates very quickly after that.

How Much Olive Oil Is Enough?

Studies which have measured the positive effects of extra virgin olive oil on health have used varying amounts of oil. Most research however has looked at the use of between 10 and 30ml a day. In many parts of the Mediterranean, as much as 70ml can be consumed by each person.

It is now known that calorie counting is not a very useful way to approach a healthy lifestyle. This is partly because different foods and diverse food combinations have a different effect on actual weight and on the tendency towards obesity which is independent of their 'calorific value'. Another contributing factor, of course, is how much exercise we get. So although olive oil is often described as being 'high in calories' this should not be a reason to avoid it! We have finally said good bye to the low fat diet.

The answer instead is the sensible consumption of an olive oil based diet with an active lifestyle. Research has shown that this way of eating helps both weight loss and the prevention of heart and other chronic diseases. Indeed it promotes good health generally. Studies have also shown that the health benefits increase with increasing amounts of extra virgin olive oil consumed. There does not appear to be a limit to this effect, but because olive oil should be enjoyed as part of a balanced and healthy diet and lifestyle, the recommended amount of extra virgin olive oil per day has settled at a minimum of two tablespoons (30ml) a day.

Summary

1 Olive oil is the everyday flavouring and most popular cooking medium in the countries of the Mediterranean basin.

2 Outside the producing countries the question 'Can I cook with extra virgin olive oil?' has been prevalent. The answer is that extra virgin olive oil is suitable for all cooking methods from slow cooking to deep fat frying.

3 There is evidence that cooking certain foods with extra virgin olive oil enhances the availability of nutrients in the food so that more are absorbed by the body than if the foods were eaten separately.

4 Marinating meat in extra virgin olive oil before cooking reduces the amount of harmful chemicals that may be produced during the cooking process.

5 Extra virgin olive oil can be used very successfully in place of hard fats such as butter and margarine in baking cakes, biscuits and pastry.

6 Extra virgin olive oil is not just a cooking medium it is also a flavouring ingredient in its own right.

7 Olive oil should not be kept in the fridge, but in a cool, dark place.

8 Current health guidelines suggest consuming a minimum of two tablespoons of extra virgin olive oil per day.

PART 3

THE OLIVE OIL DIET

OVER the years there have been many individual foods which have been described as 'superfoods' and it is certainly true that certain fruits, vegetables and berries are very rich in particular nutrients or antioxidants. However, it has been difficult to show scientifically that any single ingredient in our diet has the power to give us measurable benefits. Whether it is berries from the Himalayas or rare algae from the Pacific, the evidence for benefit is sparse and often grossly exaggerated.

Extra virgin olive oil is one of the few exceptions. It has been shown in rigorous scientific studies to have very specific health giving properties. When combined with other foods rich in beneficial nutrients and antioxidants the sum of the fusion of foods is even greater than the individual health benefits of the single ingredients alone. As the catalyst for this remarkable result, extra virgin olive oil can truly be regarded as a unique 'superfood'.

THE SEVEN PILLARS OF
THE OLIVE OIL DIET

Modern science has proved that the value which has long been attributed to olive oil was not misplaced and that the traditional dishes associated with its use are indeed particularly healthy.

The Olive Oil Diet is a way of eating every day that is not only conducive to good health but is also thoroughly enjoyable. It is not a single

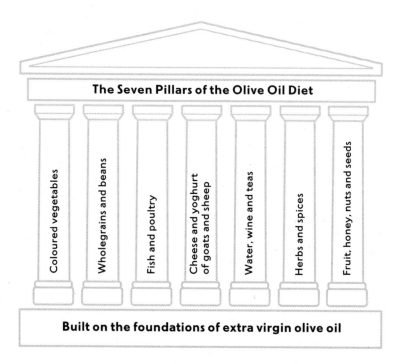

The Seven Pillars of the Olive Oil Diet

Coloured vegetables

Wholegrains and beans

Fish and poultry

Cheese and yoghurt of goats and sheep

Water, wine and teas

Herbs and spices

Fruit, honey, nuts and seeds

Built on the foundations of extra virgin olive oil

uniform pattern of eating to take up or leave when you are trying to lose weight or are not feeling too well. It is very versatile and wide ranging and can easily accommodate the seasonality and availability of particular ingredients, the varying pattern of individual tastes and preferences, and fulfil the recommended levels of extra virgin olive oil and other nutrients.

Olive oil is the foundation of this healthy way of eating with seven groups of nutritious foods based upon it. This is shown graphically in the seven pillars of the Olive Oil Diet. Olive oil is used in the preparation, cooking and flavouring of every meal and pervades the entire culinary experience. The Olive Oil Diet builds on an understanding of how olive oil works with these groups of ingredients to enhance the overall nutritional value of a meal.

Pillar 1 – Coloured Vegetables

Served raw in salads or cooked in olive oil, vegetables are an absolutely pivotal part of a healthy diet. To 'eat a rainbow' is great nutritional advice. This is because so many vitamins, minerals and antioxidants are carried in the colourful pigments of plants. The quantity and variety of vegetables consumed in the Mediterranean regions would be unimaginable without the ubiquitous presence of olive oil.

There is an additional advantage in eating a range of different vegetables at the same meal and in combining these with extra virgin olive oil. It has also been shown that combining the healthy fats in extra virgin olive oil with vegetables that are rich in nitrates, such as salads, celery, carrots and spinach, creates substances called nitro fatty acids. These have been found to lower blood pressure to a significant extent.

Ingredients
To get the best results buy as wide a variety of vegetables as you can every week, including frozen and canned vegetables.

Antioxidants in Vegetables

Phyto-nutrients can be classified by their different colours, and many have antioxidant effects which are beginning to be understood by science. Here are just a few examples.

Green: Green veggies tend to contain the antioxidant phytonutrients lutein, sulforaphanes and indoles; these include green beans, peas, celery, sprouts, green cabbage, spring greens, kale, cucumber, and many lettuces. Broccoli is perhaps the most celebrated vegetable in terms of a possible protective effect from cancers.

Red and purple: These vegetables are good sources of anthocyanin and other indole antioxidants which have been hailed as having potential to protect from us from heart disease and cancers; these include red onions, red cabbage, red peppers and aubergines.

Tomatoes are a particularly rich source of lycopene, which is being studied in relation to cancer prevention. Beetroot is rich in nitrates as well as betacyanins.

Orange and yellow: Sunny-coloured vegetables are good sources of antioxidant carotenoids; these include carrots, squashes and yellow peppers.

White: Vegetables including cauliflower, garlic, onions, parsnips and turnips are good sources of allicins, lignans and phytates. Garlic and shiitake mushrooms have been shown to have antibacterial activity which may support the immune system. Garlic also contains compounds which reduce the 'stickiness' of blood, thereby decreasing the chances of harmful blood clots forming.

Ginger: This contains gingerol, which is chemically similar to capsaicin found in chilli peppers. This antioxidant compound has also been the subject of research into anticancer properties.

Cooking vegetables with extra virgin olive oil can increase the amount of certain phytonutrients absorbed by the body from the combination. However the lower heat resistance of other phytochemicals may mean they are best eaten raw in salads and chilled soups. Avoid boiling vegetables in water. The water soluble phytonutrients will be lost in the cooking liqueur, though this can, of course, be saved and used in soups and stews. Even steaming vegetables loses some of the nutrients. The best way to cook vegetables is to poach, bake or roast in olive oil or to cook in such a way that all the cooking liqueur is absorbed back into the vegetables.

Roasting vegetables in olive oil is both easy and healthy and it is a combination which works all the year round. Open roast sliced fennel, sliced onions, broccoli or cauliflower florets or small whole kohlrabi drizzled with olive oil. Wrap whole carrots or beetroot in foil parcels with olive oil and black pepper before roasting or braise Belgian endive, leeks or fennel in a covered roasting pot with olive oil and a little home-made stock.

Vegetables to Open Roast

Here are some ideas for mixtures of vegetables to open roast with olive oil.

Caribbean mix: Choose two or three from yams, sweet potatoes, plantains, carrots, edoes, breadfruit and aubergines, flavour with chilli flakes or allspice.

Winter roots: Choose two or three from potatoes, carrots, parsnips, turnips, swede, celeriac, beetroot, kohlrabi, leeks and onions, flavour with dried sage or thyme.

Mediterranean mix: Choose two or three from red, green and yellow peppers, courgettes, aubergines, tomatoes and fennel, flavour with garlic, dried rosemary or pine nuts.

Pillar 2 – Whole Grains and Beans

Whole grains on the second pillar of the Olive Oil Diet provide low glycaemic index carbohydrates and are an important and healthy source of energy. Conversely, refined grains are detrimental to health.

Whole grains may be milled, flaked or left whole, but their outer 'husk' or bran is retained and so they are much higher in fibre than their processed equivalents. Fibre reduces the rate of absorption of sugars and reduces the risk of obesity, diabetes, high blood pressure, bowel cancer and high LDL cholesterol. As well as containing fibre whole grains contain significant amounts of vitamins, minerals and other nutrients.

Because whole grains are carbohydrates they are sometimes seen as contributors to weight gain. However this fails to differentiate unprocessed foods from the factory produced carbohydrates which dominate the food industry.

Beans or pulses are the seed of legumes. These are plants which produce their seed or fruit within a pod. They are highly nutritious, containing fibre, vitamins, minerals and antioxidants.

Ingredients

Wheat is the leading grain cereal in Europe and most of it is milled into flour or made into bread. Where possible, choose whole grain flour or wholemeal bread and pasta rather than refined white flour and white breads as these have a higher glycaemic index. For baking, use a mix of wholemeal flour and white flour. Of course, there are a few recipes which only really work well with white flour so save these dishes for special occasions.

Most pastas and couscous are made from refined wheat flour but you can buy whole grain pasta and there are other noodle products, from Japan and elsewhere, which are made with whole grain wheat flour, buckwheat or rye. Remember that wholegrain pasta will take a little longer to cook than white pasta.

Suggestions for Quick Pasta Sauces

Toss cooked pasta with any of these delicious and healthy combinations:

- a generous splash of olive oil and a handful of chopped fresh herbs

- chopped chilli peppers or garlic sautéed in olive oil

- pre-prepared basil or coriander pesto

- green or black olive paste or sundried tomato paste with more olive oil

- crushed garlic sautéed with capers and anchovies in olive oil

- crisply fried bread crumbs mixed with freshly grated Parmesan

- mixed seeds – such as sesame, pumpkin and sunflower – toasted in a dry pan, then mixed with extra virgin olive oil

Wholegrain wheat: This is used to make bulgur and cracked wheat, both of which can be used in just the same way as rice. Cracked wheat is made by drying the grains of wheat and then cracking them. Bulgur is made by boiling the grains of wheat first and then drying and cracking them. Bulgur cooks much more quickly than cracked wheat. It can also be soaked in boiling water and used without cooking.

Rice: One of the great grain staples of the world, rice, like pasta, is a natural convenience food. It may be sold as whole grain rice or, more frequently, it is polished to remove the outer husk. It is possible to find rice flakes and rice flour. Remember that brown unpolished rice takes longer to cook than white rice.

Oats: A traditional northern food and the basis for porridge, oats come in flaked form, usually known as rolled oats, and as fine, medium or coarse oatmeal. Both types use the whole grain. Beta glucan in oats can lower levels of cholesterol.

Rye and barley: Rarely used as whole grains, these are usually sold milled as flour or in flaked form. Like wholewheat grains they take a good deal of soaking to soften and even then the cooked result is very chewy. Pearl barley is the grain with the outer husks removed.

Millet: Widely used in Africa, this grain it is very easy to prepare. It comes as whole grain or in flaked form rather like rolled oats and is cooked in the same way as rice.

Buckwheat and quinoa: Although they are used in a similar way, these are not really grains at all. Buckwheat is widely used in Russia. It may be available as a raw whole grain or in a roasted form where it is known as kasha. Both forms may be cooked and served like rice or may be made into flour and used in baking. Quinoa comes in whole grain form and can be cooked in just the same way as rice or millet.

Pulses: Haricot beans, cannellini beans, butter beans, split peas and chickpeas are a good examples of pulses that a make very useful addition to fresh vegetables. They can be bought canned or dried. The former are more convenient but make sure that they have not been packed in brine or contain other additives such as preservatives. Some pulses, such as chickpeas, are ground into flour which can be used to make excellent batters (no eggs required) for deep fried vegetables and Indian specialities like onion bhajis and dosas.

Many dried pulses require soaking in water before cooking. This is because their coats do not readily absorb water in the cooking process unless they have been in contact with water for a number of hours. This is not the case for lentils, split peas and mung beans. Do not keep any pulses too long. They will go stale and will not cook properly. Do not add salt to the cooking water for legumes. This hardens them. (It is a good idea to cook more than you will need for one recipe and to freeze the rest in batches of 100–150g for use in the future.)

Many people think that peanuts are nuts but they are in fact legumes and grow underground. They combine very well with cereals like wheat to give more available protein than either ingredient on their own. This can be important in a vegetarian or vegan diet. Peanuts are often consumed as a salted snack but they are better used unsalted in savoury dishes and salads or as peanut butter in sauces such as Satay.

Pillar 3 – Fish and Poultry

Fish is a very healthy source of protein and of the Omega-3 polyunsaturated fats that are essential to us. It is important to balance the excess of Omega-6 fats which are so often found in processed foods with the regular consumption of Omega-3 polyunsaturated fats. Oily fish are higher in Omega-3s than white fish but all fish are a good source of nutrients and are relatively low in saturated fats and calories.

Poultry should be eaten more often than red meat. The white meat of poultry is generally low in saturated fat and is a good source of protein and minerals.

Ingredients

Vegetarians who do not eat any meat can find sources of healthy protein in other foods, so meat eating can be regarded as a choice.

Oily fish: This includes salmon, trout, tuna, mackerel, sardines and anchovies. Some of these fish are available in cans. These are best packed in olive oil or water rather than brine.

Shellfish and squid: These are also good sources of Omega-3. Prawns, like eggs, contain significant amounts of naturally occurring cholesterol but since the amount of cholesterol in foods is not a good indicator of LDL cholesterol in our bodies it should not be of concern. Both are healthy foods in moderation.

Fish: The environment in which a fish exists is important for health.

There have been reports of increasing levels of potentially harmful mercury in some fish, especially those sourced from contaminated areas of seas or oceans. This is a particular concern when it comes to the Mediterranean Sea. The best way to avoid eating excessive amounts of potentially harmful chemicals in fish is to vary the types of fish eaten and to sometimes choose smaller fish or shellfish – it is the larger fish higher in the food chain where such toxins are concentrated in higher quantities.

Poultry: Chicken, turkey, guinea fowl and duck as well as pheasant, wild duck and other game birds are the best choices of meat for the Olive Oil Diet. When buying farmed birds it is important to consider how the animals have been raised and what they have been eating. So-called 'battery' chickens are to be avoided.

Pot-roasting in olive oil is a great way to cook almost any bird. The dish is quick to prepare and then it can just be left to cook itself.

Pot-roasting Combinations

Try some of these delicious food combinations. Roast the ingredients in a covered pot with plenty of extra virgin olive oil and a dash of wine, vinegar or lemon juice and serve the cooking juices as a sauce.

- chicken with whole garlic cloves and lemon wedges
- guinea fowl with red pepper slices
- quail with sprigs of fresh wild marjoram
- wild duck with orange wedges
- turkey leg with garlic and black peppercorns

Red meat: There is a place for small quantities of red meat like pork, lamb and beef for those who really like it. It is important with meat to ask what your food ate. The meat of naturally reared, free roaming animals contains a much healthier proportion of fat and other nutrients than meat from animals raised in more 'industrial' methods of meat production. The latter are fed on a diet of grains rather than grazing on a mixture of plants and herbs.

Of course, meat from animals reared in this way is more expensive but smaller portions are the answer. Use the meat to add interest and flavour to a dish with plenty of vegetables and carbohydrates. Game meat is also a good choice though some cuts of venison, for example, can be quite dry and need to be marinated first and then cooked slowly. Indeed, where small quantities of red meat are included in a healthy diet, it is recommended that good quality meats are prepared with extra virgin olive oil.

Pillar 4 – Cheese and Yogurt From Goat's and Sheep's Milk

Dairy products are a great source of protein, calcium and vitamin D and are included on one of the pillars of the Olive Oil Diet. However products made from goat's or sheep's milk are recommended above those made from cow's milk. This is because they contain medium-chain rather than long-chain saturated fatty acids which do not raise harmful LDL cholesterol so much. Fermented dairy products such as these yogurts and cheeses also contain much less high glycaemic lactose. Eggs, too, are included here.

A number of traditional cheeses are still made with raw (unpasteurised) milk and they are attracting more interest and gaining in popularity, not only for their taste but also for their possible beneficial effects on health. Roquefort cheese from the south of France and some manchego cheese from Spain, both sheep's milk cheeses, are produced without the heating processes of pasteurisation. However, many soft cheeses, pasteurised or unpasteurised, are not recommended for some groups of people who may be more susceptible to infections, for example during pregnancy.

Some scientists are suggesting that the bacteria which are otherwise destroyed by the processing of cheeses might be important for our health. The populations of bacteria which naturally line our gut walls may have an influence on conditions varying from arthritis to obesity. The significance of this so called 'gut microbiome' in our intestines is beginning to be understood. The interactions between the naturally occurring microbes in our guts, those contained in foods such as fermented dairy products and the foods we eat are the subject of increasing research. Olive oil has been shown to be a very healthy part of this complex and symbiotic relationship, with a good pattern of bacteria breaking down the fats in olive oil into the particularly beneficial components.

Ingredients

Greek products such as yogurt and feta cheese were traditionally made with goat's and sheep's milk and many of the brands made in Greece itself still are. However, Greek-style yogurt, feta and halloumi cheeses produced elsewhere are often made with cow's milk. If you have to buy the latter, check that there is no added sugar. In an attempt to reduce the fat content of some dairy products, sugar has been added to enhance the taste. Such low fat products are often promoted as being healthy but in fact may not be so good for us.

Goat's and Sheep's Milk Cheese

Here are some cheeses usually made from goat and sheep's milk. Check the labels to be absolutely sure:

- Banon, Beenleigh Blue

- Cabra, Cabrales, Cacciotta, Canestrao, Cabicou, Chevre, Coleford Blue, Crottin de Chavignol

- Feta

- Halloumi

- Lanark Blue

- Malvern, Manchego

- Parmesan, Pecorino, Picos

- Ragstone, Roquefort

- Sharpham, Spenwood, St Mauré

- Vulscombe

Pillar 5 – Wine, Water and Tea

Wine is central to the culture of many regions where olive trees grow and vines and other fruit trees often stand side by side in olive groves. Wine has been celebrated for its capacity to provide health and healing for as long as olive oil. Regular consumption of a moderate amount of red wine is associated with lower rates of heart disease and stroke. Red grapes, like olives, contain polyphenolic antioxidants such as procyanidin which are passed on to the wine. These antioxidants are produced by both plants in response to stress of various kinds.

It is the antioxidants in wine which have been claimed by some to explain the so called 'French Paradox': the low rates of heart disease in France despite a diet relatively high in saturated fat. Although there is a greater emphasis on the benefits of red wine, there are many polyphenol antioxidants in white wine which are also positive for health. Of course, wine also contains alcohol which can cause harm, particularly when its breakdown product acetaldehyde increases in the blood. Drinking wine in moderation, and particularly with food, very significantly reduces the risk of harm from the alcohol content, and results in overall net benefits to health.

Liquid is important, particularly in hot climates, to prevent dehydration. Water and tea are the answer. Teas contain many different healthy compounds which have antioxidants, anti-inflammatory and antibacterial activity. This is true not only for black and green teas which contain catechins which have been shown to reduce the risk of heart disease, reduce blood pressure and cholesterol levels but also for herbal teas such as chamomile, jasmine and Greek mountain tea.

Pillar 6 – Herbs and Spices

A kitchen with a wide selection of herbs and spices will create a dining room full of flavours, reducing the need for salt to enhance taste! Add to that the diverse health properties of many herbs and spices, and every meal will also contribute to well-being. 'Hot' spices such as cinnamon, mustard and chilli are particularly rich in antioxidants as are 'earthy' spices such as fenugreek and turmeric.

Ingredients

Buy as wide as wide a range of herbs and spices as you can but bear in mind that even dried herbs do not last forever and if you are unlikely to use a particular herb or spice very much leave it out of the mix or only buy a very small amount. Most herbs and some spices can be bought fresh and if you prefer to use these keep a good selection in the fridge or freezer.

Herbs: Dried herbs are generally more potent and concentrated than fresh herbs and less will be needed. Approximately 1 teaspoon of dried herbs can be substituted for 1 tablespoon of chopped fresh herbs. Some herbs do not dry very well, losing or changing some of their flavours. These include basil, parsley and coriander leaf.

Essentials: Spices include fresh or dried chilli peppers, fresh and dried ginger, and dried pepper corns, cumin seed, coriander seed, mixed spices and a good curry powder or garam masala. Essential herbs include fresh basil, coriander and parsley, and fresh or dried thyme, rosemary, oregano, dill and tarragon.

Pillar 7 – Fruit, Honey, Nuts and Seeds

The final pillar of the Olive Oil Diet with fruit, honey, nuts and seeds offers great versatility to the diet. All these foods can be combined and used in desserts, incorporated into savoury dishes, used with breakfast porridges and muesli or simply eaten as healthy snacks.

Fruits, like vegetables, are rich sources of antioxidants. These provide protection against oxidative damage to cells and their DNA which can result in diseases including cancers. The high acidity of citrus fruits also helps to control the glycaemic index of foods following a meal. This in turn can help prevent obesity and diabetes.

Of course fruits contain sugars, often in more simple forms than the complex carbohydrates which predominate in vegetables. These simple sugars are prevented from causing sudden extreme increases in blood sugar levels by the fibrous more complex carbohydrates which make up the cell walls and other structural parts of the fruit. These compounds bind to and contain the simple sugars and reduce their absorption. In common with other fibrous plant material they also reduce absorption of cholesterol and improve bowel function.

Honey has been used for thousands of years in its raw state as a natural sweetener though it can sometimes cause illness and should be avoided for children under one year of age. Honey contains fructose and glucose as well as more complex sugars. It also contains some antioxidants in small quantities and has been shown to have some antibacterial effects.

Small amounts of honey as a natural sweetener are not considered to be harmful. However, processing of honey may involve heating to produce a clear honey and this can reduce levels of nutrients, so look for 'raw' honey or honey on the comb as the first choice,

Although some people need to avoid certain nuts because of allergies, they are an important part of the diet. They contain varying amounts of monounsaturated fats and Omega-3, vitamins, minerals and antioxidants as well as being a rich source of protein and fibre. Other people have avoided nuts because nuts, like olive oil, are relatively high in calories and so were thought to contribute to obesity. In fact, the Predimed study which demonstrated reductions in heart attacks, strokes, and overall mortality by a third with a Mediterranean style diet supplemented with additional extra virgin olive oil showed a dramatic decrease in these illnesses with a diet also enriched with nuts.

Ingredients

Fruit: To get the best results buy as wide a variety of fruit as you can every week, including frozen and dried fruits. Dried fruits add variety to the diet and only contain a little more sugar than fresh fruit.

Antioxidants in Fruit

Like vegetables, the red, blue, orange and purple pigments contained in the flesh and skins of fruit contain flavonoids, carotenoids and other polyphenolic compounds.

- **Green:** Green fruits tend to contain the antioxidant phytonutrient lutein. These include kiwi fruit, green apples, passion fruit, green figs and greengages.

- **Red and purple:** Dark fruits contain procyanidins and reservatrol. These include strawberries, raspberries, red and black currants, blackberries, plums and grapes. The longer the maceration time in wine production the higher the concentrations of these compounds which are thought to play a part in prevention of heart disease, cancers and glucose regulation.

- **Orange and yellow:** Brightly coloured fruits contain antioxidant carotenoids. Examples are include oranges, tangarines and other citrus fruits, some melons, peaches, apricots and mangoes.

- **White:** Pale fruits contain flavonoids such as quercetin; these include apples, pears, and some melons. Where practicable enjoy the skins as well.

The range of dried fruits now available is very wide, taking in apples, pears, apricots, prunes, mangoes, cranberries, raisins and sultanas. Dried fruits may need to be soaked before use. This can be done by soaking in cold water over night or in boiling water for two hours. The former method is preferable as fewer nutrients are lost into the soaking water. Check 'ready to eat' dried fruits for added sugar.

Nuts and Seeds: Including walnuts in the diet is good for the health of blood vessels, and almonds and hazelnuts have been shown to increase the feeling of fullness after eating and so reduce the risk of laying down abdominal fat. Eating them can also help to regulate blood glucose levels.

Seeds, too, are a good source of fibre, vitamins, Omega-3 and Omega-6 polyunsaturated fats and minerals such as iron, zinc, magnesium and selenium. Sesame seeds and tahini paste, which is made from finely ground sesame seeds, are excellent sources of calcium and magnesium. They also contain lignin polyphenols.

Nuts are best eaten unsalted and with their outer husks intact. Beneficial nutrients contained in the brown outer surface of almonds are lost if the nuts are 'blanched' and flaked. It is also possible to buy almonds and hazel nuts which have been ground with the husk.

Nuts and seeds with high levels of polyunsaturated fatty acids such as walnuts and sunflower seeds will deteriorate quite quickly. So buy in small quantities and do not store in the cupboard for too long.

Summary

1 The Olive Oil Diet is rich in monounsaturated fats with the addition of plenty of Omega-3 fatty acids to give a good balance with Omega-6.

2 Its carbohydrate content generally has a low glycaemic load with sweetness from honey and fruit rather than refined sugars.

3 The Olive Oil Diet is a sustainable diet made up of natural, unprocessed and mainly plant-based ingredients in balanced combinations which are rich in antioxidants.

4 The combination of ingredients in the Olive Oil Diet changes the way in which foods are absorbed and increases the availability of other beneficial nutrients.

5 This is an inclusive diet based on getting the best out of all that is eaten rather than excluding foods which are considered to be unhealthy.

6 The Olive Oil Diet offers an excellent pattern of macronutrients with good quality carbohydrates, fats and proteins together with rich quantities of micronutrients such as vitamins, minerals and plentiful antioxidants.

PUTTING THE OLIVE OIL DIET INTO PRACTICE

Even the simplest fusion of ingredients with extra virgin olive oil can be shown to be good for health. Soffritto, for example, is a classic mixture of finely chopped carrots, onions and celery gently fried in extra virgin olive oil, which is used as the base for many dishes in Italy. Slightly more elaborate, sofrito is a medley of extra virgin olive oil, garlic, tomatoes, onions and peppers used in Spain and Portugal. Both contain numerous polyphenol antioxidants with good levels of vitamins C and E.

Even more important for health are the interactions between the foods within the diet as a whole. The Olive Oil Diet is designed to give a combination of food which maximises health and protects against the harmful effects of the chemicals we are exposed to in the environment. In addition, its menu plans and recipes have been devised to make it very easy to produce meals which will naturally include the recommended two tablespoons or more of extra virgin oil every day without you really noticing it. The end result is an enjoyable way of eating which is also very healthy, delivering the benefits of the interaction of olive oil and wholesome foods.

Menu Planning

Use the Seven Pillars of the Olive Oil Diet to find inspiration for menu planning and shopping, including something from each pillar on a regular basis. Start with some simple combinations with ingredients from two or three pillars – such as coloured vegetables, fish and herbs and spices, or dairy products, fruits and seeds – to make a main dish or a group of two or three dishes. Choose items which are quick and easy to put together and move on to more complex recipes when time allows.

Add a starter, side dishes and maybe a dessert to the main dish, again choosing from the different pillars. In this way you will most likely be using foods from all the pillars of the diet and so maximising the benefits of mixing the different foods with olive oil. You will also be making wonderful meals for yourself, your family and friends.

Keeping It Simple for Every Day

Here are some ideas for combination dishes to try.

Fish and Shellfish

Eggs, prawns, mixed fresh herbs, new potatoes: Eggs made into an omelette or tortilla with the fresh herbs and prawns and diced new potatoes and fried on both sides in extra virgin olive oil.

Salmon fillets, brown rice, dill, lemon juice, coloured vegetables: Salmon is grilled and basted with a dressing made with dill, lemon juice and extra virgin olive oil. Serve on a bed of rice with the dressing drizzled over the top and mixed vegetables on the side.

Squid, lime, chilli, rocket, spinach: The squid is marinated in extra virgin olive oil with lime juice and chilli, flash-cooked on the grill and served on a salad of rocket and baby spinach leaves dressed with the lime flesh and more extra virgin olive oil.

Monkfish, prawns, fresh ginger, carrots, and spring onions with Chinese noodles: Vegetables cut into thin strips and stir-fried in extra virgin olive oil with fish and flavoured with five-spice powder then served on a bed of noodles.

Mackerel, green apples, watercress, pine nuts and lemons: The mackerel is lightly cooked and served on a bed of watercress, chopped green apples and toasted pine nuts with very thin slivers of lemon rind, dressed with extra virgin olive oil and lemon juice.

Meat

Chicken joints, spinach, watercress, walnuts and beetroot with Cajun spice mix and lemon: Chicken is fried in Cajun spices and served on a salad made up of the remaining ingredients dressed with extra virgin olive oil and white wine vinegar.

Chicken, onions, garlic, potatoes, rosemary: Small chicken pieces on the bone are open-roasted with roughly chopped onions and potatoes, topped with sprigs of rosemary and plenty of extra virgin olive oil.

Chicken breasts, mustard, tarragon, mixed root vegetables: Chicken is marinated with the mustard and tarragon in extra virgin olive oil, served baked in foil and with the open-roasted vegetables.

Small fillet steaks, butternut squash, leeks, red onions, sweet potatoes, garlic: The steak is marinated in extra virgin olive oil, mixed dried herbs and black pepper, then fried. The vegetables are diced and roasted with olive oil.

Small lamb cutlets, oranges, honey, mangetout, small French beans, new potatoes mustard: The lamb is marinated in extra virgin olive oil with orange zest, orange juice and honey, then grilled and served with the vegetables lightly stir-fried with more olive oil and new potatoes crushed with a little grainy mustard.

Vegetarian

Feta cheese, red and green peppers, cucumber, tomatoes, lemon juice: Salad made with chopped vegetables and dressed with lemon juice and extra virgin olive oil and topped with feta cheese and fresh marjoram.

Chickpeas, spinach, baby sweet corn, tomatoes: The chickpeas are soaked overnight and placed with the other vegetables and canned tomatoes in a slow cooker with extra virgin olive oil. On a low setting, the dish is ready by dinner time.

Roquefort cheese, chicory, pea shoots, walnuts, sherry vinegar: The Roquefort cheese is crumbled over a salad of chicory spears, pea shoots and walnuts dressed with extra virgin olive oil and a little sherry vinegar.

Fennel, red onions, small chicory spears, garlic, flaked almonds, Greek yogurt: The fennel and onion are sliced and roasted on a tray with chicory spears cut in half lengthways, whole garlic cloves and almonds all drizzled with plenty of extra virgin olive oil and served with a sharp Greek yogurt.

Rocket and mixed leaves, Parmesan cheese, hazelnuts, sundried tomatoes, dried figs: The salad leaves are topped with shavings of Parmesan cheese, toasted hazelnuts and strips of sundried tomatoes and chopped figs. The dish is dressed with extra virgin olive oil mixed with a good balsamic vinegar.

Desserts and sweet foods

The last pillar of the Olive Oil Diet points the way to healthy dessert choices. Fresh fruits make very quick and easy desserts and, of course, numerous studies have shown the benefits of eating several pieces of fruit every day.

The choice of fresh fruits on sale today is vast, and berries and other fruit can also be bought frozen for when the fresh are out of season. A mixture of fruit, perhaps with some ewe's or goat's yogurt is a delicious way to end, or even start, the day.

Making Fruit Desserts with Olive Oil

- **Sliced fruit platters:** Choose your fruit and dress with a splash of extra virgin olive oil and some fresh herbs or a pinch of spice. For extra speed use a flavoured olive oil. Here are some suggestions:

    Oranges with rosemary and honey
    Pineapple with finely sliced root ginger and a pinch of cinnamon
    Kiwi fruit and strawberries with mint
    Pears and mangoes with toasted chopped nuts

- **Grilled fruit kebabs:** Marinate the fruit in a mixture of extra virgin olive oil, fruit juice and a little honey. Cook under the grill in winter and on the barbecue in the summer. Make up combinations from any of the following fruit: banana chunks, apricot halves, pears cut into wedges, strawberries, kiwi fruit cut into quarters, melon balls and pineapple chunks.

- **Oven-baked fruits:** Add a splash of olive oil and bake for about 10–15 minutes in a hot oven. This method is particularly useful when soft fruits simply refuse to ripen. Nuts, seeds and whole grains can be combined to make excellent crumble toppings.

Chocolate: The good news for chocoholics is that a small amount of dark chocolate is consistent with the Olive Oil Diet. It has been shown that due to its balance of saturated and monounsaturated fats, cocoa does not raise cholesterol levels. It also contains plenty of antioxidants. Thus chocolate with very high percentages of cocoa is not as unhealthy as may be thought at first glance.

Snacks and Nibbles

So many snack foods have a great deal of salt in them and a whole range of other ingredients which have no nutritional value. Here are some ideas for snack foods which are not full of salt or sugar.

- a 30g handful of unsalted nuts
- mixed nuts and seeds
- crunchy vegetable cruditées
- cherry tomatoes
- mixed dried fruits
- green and black olives
- a banana, apple or pear

Breakfast

Wholegrain breakfast cereals with no additives, plain oat porridge and muesli made with oats, wholegrain cereals, nuts and dried or fresh fruit all make very healthy breakfasts. When time allows, you might choose to add wholemeal fruit muffins, toasted soda bread, banana pancakes or French toast, all made with olive oil, to the breakfast menu.

In the olive oil producing regions, the traditional breakfast is composed of extra virgin olive oil drizzled over toasted bread, maybe with a rubbing of tomato, garlic or even honey and a perhaps a slab of goat's cheese on the side.

Weekly Menus

A typical weekly main meal menu plan to serve at lunch or dinner might include a variety of vegetable dishes such as soups, pasta and rice with eggs, cheese and yogurt; two main meals based on fish and two on poultry, limiting red meat to one meal or less.

The best plan is to be as wide ranging and imaginative as possible. There is no need to stick to the old 'meat and two veg' pattern. Two or three dishes of equal weight can make a very attractive meal. Think of the meat and fish ingredients as flavouring ingredients rather than as the main star of the meal. Nor is it necessary to cook every part of every dish. Grilled meats and fish are both good served on a bed of salad leaves or raw vegetables. Fresh fruit, too, can be used in hot and cold savoury dishes.

Here are some menus built up from recipes in the Recipes for Well-being section.

Vegetarian Menus
– Warm Salad of Mixed Grilled Vegetables (see page 181)
– Greek Cheese Fritters with Beetroot Medley (see page 223)
– Maids of Honour (see page 257)

– Pecorino Salad with Fruit and Olives (see page 194),
– Cavatelli with Broad Beans and Peas (see page 222)
– Yogurt with thyme and honey

- Soupe au Pistou (see page 205) with Sprouted Soda Bread (see page 266)
- Braised Pears with Ginger and Raisins (see page 254)

- Egg Pilaf (see page 164) served with Curried Lentils (see page 168) and a tomato salad
- Fresh fruit salad
- Three-fruit Salad (see page 185)
- Spinach-wrapped Nut Roast with Chilli Yogurt Salsa (see page 228) with braised chicory
- Grilled Fruit Kebabs (see page 134)

Vegan Menus
- Grapefruit and Avocado Salad with Fresh Herbs (see page 173)
- Penne with Broccoli Pesto (see page 220)
- Sliced fruit platter (see page 134)

- Three-fruit Salad (see page 185)
- Lebanese Aubergine Casserole (see page 226) with Coriander Bulgur (see page 241)
- Date and Banana Cookies (see page 272)

Fish and Seafood Menus
- Celery and Tomato Soup with Parsley (see page 204)
- Spicy Seafood Stir-fry with Noodles (see page 229)
- Apricots with Sesame Crumble (see page 256)

- Stuffed and Grilled Little Gem Lettuces (see page 213)
- Salmon with Ginger and Spring Onions on a Bed of Chard (see page 237)
- Strawberries and Greek yogurt

- Herring and Beetroot Salad (see page 180), Tuna and Green Bean Salad (see page 193) with chicory and watercress and a green salad to fit
- Fried Bananas with Mixed Seeds (see page 251)

- Tossed green salad with olive oil vinaigrette
- Tuna with Garlic and Chilli Beans (see page 231)
- Profiteroles (see page 259)

Meat Menus
- Fig and Black Olive Tapenade with Rocket Salad (see page 183) and Oatcakes (see page 275)
- Fried Chicken on Warm Quinoa Salad (see page 177) with apricots, pickled lemons and a green salad
- Dates and sliced oranges

- Lamb Cutlets with Spiced Beetroot (see page 246)
- Slice of Carrot Cake (see page 260)

- Chickpea Broth with Coriander (see page 201) and Parmesan Toasts
- Lamb Cutlets with Lemon Dill Potatoes and Broccoli with Red Peppers and Hazelnuts
- Banana Pancakes (see page 253)

Adding More Extra Virgin Olive Oil to the Menu

Here are some easy and enjoyable ways to boost your intake of extra virgin olive oil:

- serve a robust oil with strips of carrot and cucumber as dippers before the meal

- drizzle oil over bread rolls or toast instead of serving bread and butter at lunch or dinner

- drizzle on toast with a little honey for breakfast

- leave the bottle of oil on the table to add as a condiment to soups, pasta, stews and vegetables

- fill a hip flask with oil to take with you to dress desk-top lunches or when you eat out

SHOPPING FOR THE
HEALTHIEST INGREDIENTS

PLANNING ahead makes shopping easier and quicker and removes the temptation to pop a quick ready-meal into the basket when you are busy. Whether you like to shop on the day or get all the shopping out of the way at the weekend, think about the meal or meals you are going to serve, keeping the image of the Seven Pillars of the Olive Oil Diet in mind. This will help you to see good combinations which might be on offer that day.

Fresh Food

Fresh is best for extra virgin olive oil and it is also best for a wide range of other ingredients, particularly fruit and vegetables. Achieving this is not always so easy. The food chain can be a very long one and food grown thousands of miles from home may be quite old before it reaches the shops. Even locally grown salad ingredients, such as lettuce and watercress, can take a few days to reach the supermarket shelves. In some instances losses of up to 45 per cent of the vitamin C content have been recorded from harvesting vegetables to placing them on the table. Watch out, too, for nutrient loss in salad vegetables presented in controlled atmosphere packs. This method of packaging can reduce the amount of nutrients in the leaves and you may not be getting as much vitamin C and other nutrients as you think.

Of course, in our modern world food can be preserved by freezing and canning. There is no evidence to suggest that freezing fresh vegetables, for example, is harmful or reduces their nutritional quality. Indeed, because of the time factor, some products – such as frozen peas – are a good deal 'fresher' when they are frozen than 'fresh' peas in the shops. Frozen products also have the advantage of offering just as much as you want at any one time with no wastage. Canned products, too, can be as healthy as their fresh equivalent. However, a good many manufacturers add salt or sugar for flavour or in order to increase shelf life, so it is important to check the labels for these and other additives.

A wide variety of foods from across the world is often available at all times of year. Green beans are imported to the UK from Africa and mangoes from South America. Strawberries are on sale in the winter. This choice can be attractive but the long distances can cause problems. Fruits often do not ripen properly and flavours are not always very good. Buying seasonal, local produce is, of course, a personal choice, often made for reasons of protecting the environment, sustaining local farmers and markets or preserving unique varieties.

Whilst organic foods may be more expensive, there is some evidence that they may be richer in antioxidants and they will not contain pesticides or other chemical residues.

Ready-made Foods

Ready-made and processed foods have become a part of life for busy people. They range from items like tomato passata, guacamole and olive pastes – which offer short cuts to more interesting dishes – through sauces, pasta dishes, casseroles, bakes, pizzas and cakes to complete meals in a box. But these foods are often full of salt, sugar and refined cereals. They may also contain ingredients which have no nutritional value that are included simply to increase the shelf life or to enhance the taste. These added substances can do harm and actually reduce the likelihood of gaining most benefit from the healthy natural ingredients in the foods.

On the whole, is it is advisable to stick to ingredients that are not packaged or processed into 'ready' food for convenience or for presentation. Labelling laws have made it easier to understand what is in our foods, but it is also clear that cooking from scratch, combining natural and identifiable produce to create a meal is the best way to be sure of the purity of the foods we eat.

However, having to make everything from scratch is difficult for many and very time-consuming. If you look carefully you can find some very good ready-made foods in the shops and the range is increasing as small food companies come into the market, competing on the basis of their lack of additives and potentially harmful ingredients.

Start by making a point of always checking the label and reading the list of ingredients before you buy. Look to see if the product is free from preservatives and artificial flavourings. Assess the added salt and sugar levels and avoid ingredients like stabilisers and emulsifiers which are not adding to the nutritional value of the food. Other ingredients to look out for and avoid include caramel, corn syrup, fructose, dextrose and maltose, all of which denote added sugar.

Get to know the brands which fulfil these criteria and look out for other products in their range which you might like.

Ready-made Foods Worth Looking Out For

Here are some ideas for ready-made items which are time-consuming to make at home, but which can be particularly useful in speeding up preparation and adding interest to dishes.

Curry sauces: There are a number of ready-made sauces with no additives which are designed to give an authentic curry flavour to which you can add your own fresh ingredients.

Filo pastry: This very thin and crispy pastry is very difficult to make but very easy to use. In the Western diet, pastry has become synonymous with high calories and poor-quality processed food. However, filo pastry made with extra virgin olive oil is healthy and delicious.

Houmous: Houmous is made from ground chickpeas, which are rich in antioxidants and fibre. They are often mixed with tahini or sesame cream and garlic. This makes a good dip but it can also be used to stuff baked vegetables or to bind nut and vegetable patties and roasts.

Guacamole: Guacamole is made from pureéed avocado pears mixed with garlic, herbs and sometimes tomatoes. Avocados are rich in oleic acid, fibre and potassium. Guacamole makes a good dip but can also be used to stuff raw vegetable canapés or spread on snacks and canapés.

Olive pastes: Crushed olives may be mixed with a variety of other ingredients, such as lemon, herbs, garlic, capers or dried tomatoes. Anchoiade is a paste made with olive, capers and anchovies. Spread on toast or bread these pastes make a good appetiser or snack. Alternatively use them as a base for pasta sauces.

Passata: Passata is a purée of fresh, uncooked, or sometimes cooked, tomatoes which have had the skin and seeds removed. It makes a great base for pasta sauces and tomato sauces of all kinds. Use to moisten baked vegetables and in stews and casseroles.

Pesto: Pesto is a paste made of finely chopped basil, garlic, Parmesan cheese and pine nuts. It makes a good pasta sauce. It can also be used to add piquancy to soups and casseroles. Add when the dish is served.

Nut roasts: There are some good dry nut roast mixes with no additives to which you can add your own fresh vegetables.

Ready-made Foods to Avoid

'Convenience' foods, even when promoted as being healthy, are often very high in sugar or salt.

Breakfast cereals and some oats preparations: In theory, a low GI mix of wholegrain cereals, oats, nuts and dried fruit produces a very healthy breakfast. However, many packaged breakfast cereals have added sugars and salt. Even simple porridge products are often sweetened.

Concentrated fruit juices: Although these would seem to be very healthy products, the sugar content is very high and the fibre content is very low.

Sugar: Avoid adding sugar to drinks. People are often surprised how quickly they get used to tea and coffee without sugar. There is no need to use sugar in desserts or baking where fresh fruit, home-made fruit purées and a little honey can do the job just as well.

Smoothies: High-sugar drinks and so-called smoothies are best avoided as both have very high concentrations of sugar.

Processed meats: Pies and sausages which might contain mechanically recovered meat are to be avoided. Other processed meats, such as bacon and ham, have been implicated in possible increased heart disease and bowel cancer. One theory is that the sodium nitrite commonly used as a preservative in the curing process may be harmful. More recently the World Health Organisation has warned against processed meats on the basis of their cancer-forming properties.

Stock cubes and ready-made sauces: The salt content in these products can be very high, so check the label.

Processed foods: Processed foods are often very high in refined sugar and carbohydrates, such as pizzas, bought cakes and biscuits and most ready-meals.

Fat spreads: Fat spreads such as margarine, even those with added 'functional' chemicals or claims to reduce weight, are very high in poly-unsaturated fatty acids and add to the imbalance of Omega-6 and Omega-3 fatty acids in the diet.

PART 4

RECIPES FOR WELL-BEING

THE Olive Oil Diet is a diet without borders. Many of the recipes and ideas included in this section of the book have been inspired by the flavours and traditional cuisines of the areas where the olive tree grows. But many have come from totally different backgrounds, drawing the use of olive oil into a much wider context than just that of the Mediterranean. The Olive Oil Diet should not be regarded as a restrictive regional diet. Curries, pilafs, salsas and noodle dishes all fall happily into the healthy versatility of the Diet. The nutritional principles of the Olive Oil Diet can be applied to world cuisine as a whole.

Notes on the Recipes

- All the recipes use extra virgin olive oil as the cooking medium and often as the flavouring ingredient as well. Since we always recommend offering extra virgin olive oil as a condiment, it is assumed you will have a bottle on the table and is not listed in every recipe.

- The use of salt has been kept to a minimum, being specified only where really necessary, and sugar is not used at all. Refined cereals are also kept to a minimum.

- All the recipes have been tested and a fan oven was used for those recipes in which an oven is needed.

- All recipes are designed for four people unless otherwise stated.

- Use medium eggs, fruit and vegetables.

- Spoon measurements are level.

SNACKS AND LIGHT MEALS

ITALIAN SAGE TOASTS

This is a quick snack to make and it disappears in seconds! You can use any kind of cheese from goat's cheese log to buffalo mozzarella – the choice is yours.

Serves 2

4 slices bread
1 large egg, beaten
50ml extra virgin olive oil
100g cheese, sliced
2 small sprigs fresh sage

1 Dip the slices of bread in the beaten egg.
2 Heat the olive oil and fry until just beginning to cook on one side.
3 Turn over two of the cooked slices and top with slices of cheese and sage. Then with the remaining slices, put them fried-side down on the cheese.
4 Continue frying until the first side of the bread is browned. Turn the whole sandwiches over and brown the other side.
5 Serve at once.

AVOCADO AND FETA TOASTS

Avocados served with a good extra virgin olive oil vinaigrette, perhaps with a little finely chopped red onion, make excellent snacks in their own right. This is another way of serving them for a change.

Serves 4

4 large slices bread
1 avocado, stoned and peeled
juice of ½ small lemon
2–3 spring onions, finely chopped
125g feta cheese, crumbled
60ml extra virgin olive oil, plus extra for serving

1 Toast the bread.

2 Mash the avocado flesh with a fork, then stir in the lemon juice and spring onions.

3 Spread this mixture over the slices of toast. Top with the crumbled feta cheese and drizzle with olive oil.

4 Place under a hot grill for 2–3 minutes and serve at once with more olive oil on the side.

AUBERGINE BRUSCHETTA

This is a variation on the more traditional bruschetta made with tomatoes, basil and garlic.

Serves 4

2 tsp pine kernels
2 tsp sunflower seeds
3 tbsp olive oil, plus extra for brushing
1 garlic clove, peeled and crushed
2 tsp sundried tomato paste
1 small aubergine, diced
3 small tomatoes, coarsely chopped
2 tablespoons chopped fresh parsley
salt and freshly ground black pepper
4 slices French country bread or/ Ciabatta (opened lengthwise)
For the garnish
8–12 small black olives
a few sprigs fresh parsley

1 Toast the pine kernels and sunflower seeds under the grill or in a dry frying pan until lightly browned.

2 Heat the olive oil and fry the garlic until softened, then stir in the sundried tomato paste and add the aubergine. Cook for 8–12 minutes until just tender but do not allow it to go mushy.

3 Add the tomatoes and parsley, season with salt and pepper and cook for a couple of minutes until hot.

4 Meanwhile brush the bread with the extra olive oil and toast on both sides.

5 Spread the toast with the aubergine mixture. Sprinkle with the

prepared nuts and seeds. Garnish with black olives and sprigs of fresh parsley. Drizzle with more oil if necessary.

Healthy Highlight

The combination of the extra virgin olive oil, garlic and aubergine creates a rich and powerful blend of antioxidants. The anti-inflammatory sulphur compounds in garlic and the anthocyanins in the deep purple pigment of the aubergine soak up the goodness of the oil.

SPANISH SCRAMBLED EGGS

This is scrambled eggs with a difference. Known simply as *revuelta* in Andalucia, the eggs are scrambled with a mixture of vegetables. It's a great way to use up small quantities of leftover vegetables.

Serves 4

3 tbsp extra virgin olive oil
1 onion, peeled and very finely chopped
1 garlic clove (optional), peeled and chopped
1 stick celery, very finely chopped
4 tbsp canned baby broad beans or cooked green beans, chopped
2 small tomatoes, seeded and chopped
6 eggs, beaten
2 tbsp water
1 tbsp chopped fresh parsley
1 knob of butter
salt and freshly ground black pepper

To serve

crusty wholemeal or farmhouse bread

1 Heat 2 tablespoons of the olive oil in a pan and add the onion and garlic, if using. Sauté gently for 2–3 minutes. Do not allow to brown.

2 Add all the remaining vegetables and continue cooking and stirring for another 3–4 minutes.

3 Meanwhile, beat the eggs with the water and the remaining olive oil, and season with pepper. Melt the butter in a separate pan and lightly scramble the eggs, stirring gently until only just set.

4 Just before serving, stir in the cooked vegetable mixture and parsley.

5 Serve at once with crusty wholemeal or farmhouse bread.

TUNA SALAD IN A BUN

This substantial snack is known as *pan bagnat* in the south of France, where it originates. Any kind of flat teacakes or bread rolls can be used, but you may need to adjust the quantities of the filling to fit the size.

Serves 2

2 large wholemeal bread rolls, split in half
2–3 tbsp extra virgin olive oil
a few soft lettuce leaves
1 tomato, sliced
160g can tuna in olive oil, drained and flaked
1 red onion, peeled and thinly sliced
½ small red pepper, seeded and cut into rings
12 black olives, pitted
1 hard-boiled egg, sliced (optional)

1 Brush each split half of the buns with olive oil.

2 Place the bases on a board and arrange the lettuce leaves and tomato slices so that all the bread is covered. Next add the tuna and onion and pepper rings, adding more olive oil to taste.

3 Finish with the black olives and egg, if using. Place the second half of the bun on top and press down well together.

4 Serve at once.

MUSHROOMS WITH SPINACH AND POACHED EGGS

This method of slow cooking the eggs in olive oil is akin to poaching the eggs. You can serve with crusty wholemeal rolls to mop up the juices, if you like.

Serves 2

4 large Portobello or field mushrooms
100ml extra virgin olive oil
200g frozen chopped spinach, thawed and drained
1 heaped tbsp Greek yogurt
freshly ground black pepper
freshly grated nutmeg
2 eggs

1 Heat the grill and brush the mushrooms all over with 1 tablespoon olive oil, making sure that there is plenty in the gills. Place under the grill and cook for about 3–4 minutes on each side.

2 Meanwhile heat the spinach in a pan until hot, then stir in the yogurt, black pepper and nutmeg.

3 Gently heat the remaining olive oil in a frying pan and break in the

eggs. As the whites of the egg spread, fold them over the yolk and continue cooking very gently for about 4 minutes. The oil should not bubble and the yolk should remain really runny.

4 To serve, place 2 mushrooms close together on each serving plate and top with spinach, then an egg. Serve at once.

AUBERGINE FRITTERS WITH BAGNA CAUDA

These lovely crispy fritters are made with chickpea or chana flour which can be purchased at most Indian and Middle Eastern grocers. The advantage of this flour is that you do not need to use egg. However, if you cannot find any chana flour you could use an ordinary milk, egg and white flour batter.

Serves 2

3 tbsp chana flour
4 tbsp water
4 tbsp extra virgin olive oil
1 medium to large aubergine, cut into 8 slices
For the bagna cauda
100ml extra virgin olive oil
2 garlic cloves, peeled and crushed
4 anchovy fillets, finely chopped
4 tbsp chopped fresh mixed herbs
freshly ground black pepper

1 Start by making the *bagna cauda*. Gently heat the olive oil in a saucepan and blend in the garlic and anchovy fillets. Do not allow the oil to get too hot.

2 To make the aubergine fritters, mix the chana flour and water to make a smooth, thick cream.

3 Heat the olive oil in a frying pan.

4 Dip the slices of aubergine in the chana batter to coat well. Drop into the hot olive oil and fry on both sides for about 3–4 minutes until they are crisp and golden and the aubergine is cooked through.

5 Add the herbs and black pepper to the *bagna cauda* and spoon over the aubergine to serve.

CURRIED TOMATOES ON HOMEMADE CHUTNEY TOAST

This is a very good way of giving more flavour to winter tomatoes. Remember, the riper the tomatoes the faster they will cook.

Serves 4

4 tbsp extra virgin olive oil

6 tomatoes

1 ½ tsp mild, medium or strong curry powder to taste

1 tsp ground cumin

1 tsp ground coriander

6 slices wholemeal bread

6 heaped tsp homemade chutney (see pages 157–158)

1 Heat the olive oil in a large non-stick frying pan.

2 Cut the tomatoes in half horizontally and place skin-side down in the hot oil. Sprinkle with the curry powder and spices.

3 Cook the tomatoes over a medium heat for about 10–15 minutes,

turning from time to time to release the juice from the tomatoes and to cook them evenly.

4 Toast the bread, then spread each slice with a teaspoonful of chutney. Arrange on plates and top with six tomato halves each.

MANGO CHUTNEY

Chutney is an excellent ingredient for a number of interesting recipes but commercial chutneys are full of added sugar. This recipe has no added sugar or salt.

Makes 2 x 300g jars

75g dried mangoes
1 tbsp extra virgin olive oil
1 large onion, peeled and finely chopped
2 eating apples, cored and diced
50g raisins
100ml cider vinegar
2 tbsp good-quality balsamic vinegar of Modena
½ tsp allspice
¼ tsp ground ginger
¼ tsp cayenne pepper
1 clove

1 Place the dried mangoes in a basin and just cover with boiling water. Leave to stand for 2 hours until softened.

2 Heat the olive oil in a frying pan and gently fry the onion until slightly softened.

3 Drain the mangoes, reserving the water, then chop. Add to the onion with the soaking water. Add all the remaining ingredients.

4 Bring the mixture to the boil, reduce the heat and cover with a lid. Simmer for about 45 minutes until the mixture is beginning to thicken. Stir from time to time to prevent the chutney sticking to the base of the pan.

5 Remove the lid and boil off any remaining liquid over a high heat, stirring all the time.

6 Remove from the heat and leave to cool, uncovered.

7 Store in sterilised jam jars and use as required. It will last for 6 months stored in a cool dry place. Once opened, store in the fridge and use within 3 months.

Suggestion

For a sweeter chutney, add ½ small pineapple, well chopped, instead of one of the apples.

GREEN TOMATO AND DATE CHUTNEY

This is another chutney which is very easy to make at home.

Makes 3 x 300g jars

1kg green tomatoes
2 eating apples, cored and quartered
2 onions, peeled and quartered
100g pitted dates
2 tbsp extra virgin olive oil
100ml cider vinegar
4 tbsp good-quality balsamic vinegar of Modena
½ tsp mustard seed

½ tsp cayenne pepper

1 pinch allspice

1 Place the tomatoes in a blender with the apples, onions and dates and process until well chopped.

2 Heat the olive oil in a pan, add the chopped mixture and cook for 5 minutes over a medium heat.

3 Add the vinegars and spices. Return to the boil and simmer for about 1 hour until the mixture thickens, stirring from time to time to stop it sticking to the pan.

4 Remove from the heat and leave to cool.

5 Store in sterilised jam jars. It will last for 6 months stored in a cool dry place. Once opened, store in the fridge and use within 3 months.

VEGETABLE AND NUT BURGERS WITH GREEK PICKLED VEGETABLES

You can ring the changes on these vegetable patties by using different combinations of nuts and herbs. Start with the soffritto of onion, carrot and celery and stir it into the mashed beans. Then add the nuts and flavourings of your choice. You can use canned beans or soak and cook dried beans in advance.

Serves 4

3 tbsp extra virgin olive oil

1 small onion, peeled and finely chopped

1 small carrot, peeled and finely chopped

1 stick celery, finely chopped

2 garlic cloves, peeled and crushed

100g cooked white beans, such as cannellini, haricot, butter or gigantas
50g ground nuts
1 bunch watercress
2 eggs, beaten
50g dried breadcrumbs
25g Parmesan cheese, freshly grated
plenty of freshly ground black pepper
To serve
Greek Pickled Vegetables (see page 161)

1 Place 1 tablespoon of olive oil in a frying pan, add the onion, carrot, celery and garlic and fry gently over a low heat. Do not allow the mixture to brown.

2 Transfer to a food processor, add the beans and process to make a thick paste. Next add the nuts and watercress and blend again. If the mixture is very wet, add some more nuts.

3 Shape into small burgers using two tablespoons. Chill and keep on one side until required.

4 Put the eggs in a shallow bowl and mix the breadcrumbs and Parmesan in a second shallow bowl. Dip each vegetable burger in beaten egg, then in the Parmesan and breadcrumb mixture, making sure that they are well coated.

5 To cook, heat the remaining olive oil in a frying pan and fry the burgers on each side for about 3 minutes until well browned.

Variation

Use fresh raw spinach with a handful of parsley instead of watercress.

GREEK PICKLED VEGETABLES

This method of lightly pickling can be used for most vegetables. I have chosen a very basic winter mix but you could use courgettes, cucumbers, mushrooms, garlic cloves or whatever else you have to hand. If you choose quick-cook vegetables, do not add them to the mix until the second stage.

Makes 2 × 420g jars

200g cauliflower florets, taken off the main stalk
125g carrots, peeled and sliced
14–16 small or pickling onions, peeled
2 sticks celery
4 small long sweet green peppers
150ml extra virgin olive oil
100ml white wine vinegar
50ml fresh lemon juice
a few black peppercorns
2 bay leaves
1 sprig fresh thyme

1 Place the prepared vegetables in a large pan and barely cover with water. Bring to the boil and boil quite rapidly for 10 minutes.

2 Remove the vegetables from the cooking liquor and keep on one side. Fast-boil the liquid to reduce to 400ml.

3 Return the vegetables to the pan with all the remaining ingredients and return to the boil. Reduce the heat and cover with a lid. Simmer for a further 10 minutes.

4 Remove from the heat and leave to cool.

5 Transfer the vegetables to sterilised jars and fill up with some of the pickling liquor. Store in the fridge for up to 2 months.

OVEN-BAKED FRITTATA WITH CRISPY BROCCOLI

Serve with crusty bread drizzled with olive oil.

Serves 4

6 tbsp extra virgin olive oil
1 small onion, peeled and finely chopped
1 red pepper, seeded and cut into thin strips
4 eggs, beaten
100g soft goat's cheese
4 tbsp milk
150g tenderstem broccoli, trimmed
freshly ground black pepper

1 Preheat the oven to 180°C/gas 4.

2 Spoon half the oil into a 22cm ovenproof flan dish and add the onion and pepper. Stir to coat them in the oil. Cook in the oven for 5–6 minutes, stirring once.

3 Mix the beaten eggs with the soft cheese and milk and season with pepper. Pour over the onions and peppers.

4 Place the flan dish on a baking tray and arrange the tenderstem broccoli on the tray at the side. Drizzle with the rest of the olive oil.

5 Bake for 10–12 minutes until the frittata is set in the middle and the broccoli is lightly browned and crisp.

Suggestions

Use peas, chopped green beans or asparagus or any combination of these in place of the peppers.

Use feta cheese for a sharper flavour.

FILO TART WITH PEPPERS

If you don't like anchovies, simply leave them out and use whole green or black olives instead.

Serves 4

5–6 tbsp extra virgin olive oil, plus extra for greasing
2 large green peppers, seeded and cut into quarters
2 large red peppers, seeded and cut into quarters
6 sheets filo pastry
1 large beef tomato, sliced
2–4 spring onions, sliced
115g soft goat's cheese with no rind
1 × 50g can anchovy fillets
freshly ground black pepper

1 Preheat the oven to 180°C/gas 4 and lightly grease a 36cm × 26cm baking tray.

2 Line a second baking tray with foil and place the pepper quarters skin-side up on the foil. Bake in the oven for about 20 minutes until the skins begin to blacken.

3 Remove the skins from the peppers, then cut the flesh into a few smaller pieces and keep on one side.

4 Place a sheet of filo pastry on the prepared baking tray, brush with olive oil, then place another sheet on top. Continue to use all the pastry, brushing each layer with plenty of olive oil as you go.

5 Make 5 rows of vegetables across the pastry: red pepper, green pepper, tomatoes, green pepper, then red pepper.

6 Sprinkle on the spring onions and dot with teaspoonfuls of goat's cheese. Arrange the anchovies over the top and season generously with pepper.

7 Brush with more olive oil and bake for 10–12 minutes until the pastry is brown and crispy underneath. Cut into quarters to serve.

EGG PILAF

The inspiration for this recipe came from Madeira and the best bananas to use are the small sweet bananas from that island, if you can find them, although any bananas will do. Serve with sliced tomatoes dressed with extra virgin olive oil, lime juice and chilli.

Serves 4

100g long-grain rice
200ml water
3 tbsp extra virgin olive oil
6–8 whole pimento or allspice seeds
1 large onion, peeled and finely chopped
6 large hard-boiled eggs, roughly chopped
4 tbsp cooked peas
3 tbsp flaked almonds, toasted in a dry pan
4 small ripe bananas or 2 large ones, peeled and sliced
2 tbsp sultanas
salt and freshly ground black pepper

1 Place the rice and water in a pan, bring to the boil, then cook for 12–15 minutes until the rice is cooked through and all the liquid has been absorbed. These quantities will make 300g cooked rice.

2 Heat the olive oil in a wok and fry the whole pimento seeds for 1 minute, then crush with a wooden spoon. Add the onion and fry until well browned.

3 Add the cooked rice and toss well with the onion. Stir in the chopped eggs. Next add all the remaining ingredients and stir-fry over a medium heat for a further 2–3 minutes until thoroughly heated through.

Suggestion

Use toasted and chopped pistachio nuts in place of the flaked almonds.

QUICK BLUE CHEESE AND BROCCOLI SOUFFLÉ

Soufflés always sound as though they will be difficult to make but this is ease itself.

Serves 2

50g tenderstem broccoli, finely chopped
2 shallots, peeled and finely chopped
1 tbsp extra virgin olive oil
100g Roquefort cheese, crumbled
4 eggs
2 tbsp milk

1 Preheat the oven to 180°C/gas 4.
2 Mix the chopped broccoli with the shallots in the base of a 10cm deep ovenproof dish. Pour on the olive oil and stir the vegetables together in the oil. Bake for 5–6 minutes.
3 Meanwhile, mix all the remaining ingredients in a basin, making sure that the pieces of cheese are broken down and well blended with the

eggs and milk. Pour this mixture over the vegetables and return the dish to the oven.

4 Bake for 18–20 minutes until well fluffed up and cooked in the centre.

Suggestion

Use cauliflower florets in place of broccoli.

VEGETABLE FILO FLAN

This filo flan is good hot or cold and once again it can be served as a light lunch or as a first course at a grand meal.

Serves 4

4 sheets filo pastry
75ml extra virgin olive oil, plus extra for greasing
225g courgettes
6 eggs, beaten
3 tbsp milk
3 tomatoes, peeled, seeded and diced
1 green pepper, seeded and finely diced
125g hard goat's or ewe's milk cheese, grated

1 Preheat the oven to 200°C/gas 6 and grease a 20cm loose-based cake tin.

2 One at a time, brush the sheets of filo pastry with olive oil and place in the cake tin so that the corners extend over the side. Turn the tin each time so the points go around the edge like the spokes on a wheel.

3   Steam the courgettes in a steamer or in a very little water for about 8 minutes until just tender. Drain well, then slice.

4   Heat 1 tablespoon olive oil in a small pan. Mix together the eggs and milk, add to the pan and lightly scramble. Stir in the tomatoes and pepper.

5   Layer the egg mixture with the cheese and courgettes in the flan tin. When it is full, fold the filo pastry corners over the top to seal and pour over any remaining olive oil.

6   Bake for 25 minutes until crisp and golden.

7   Leave to cool slightly, then serve cut into wedges.

VEGETABLE TORTILLA WITH MINCED BEEF

This is not only a very quick and easy dish to cook, it is also very versatile. You can use any vegetables that you happen to have to hand and there's no need to add the meat if you are a vegetarian. Serve with a tomato salad dressed with olive oil, lemon juice and spring onions.

Serves 2

4 tbsp extra virgin olive oil
2–3 sticks celery, chopped
2 potatoes, peeled and diced
½ red pepper, seeded and chopped
1 onion, peeled and chopped
1 courgette, diced
100g minced beef
1 tbsp chopped fresh coriander
2 eggs, beaten
1 tbsp milk

1 Heat the olive oil in a frying pan and add all the chopped and diced vegetables except the courgette. Fry over a medium heat for 5 minutes, keeping the vegetables on the move with a spatula.

2 Stir in the diced courgette and the minced beef and continue cooking for about 10–15 minutes until the potatoes are almost cooked through. Stir from time to time.

3 Sprinkle the coriander over the top. Mix together the egg and milk and pour into the pan. Turn up the heat a little and cook for a further 2–3 minutes on each side, turning the tortilla over like a pancake.

Suggestions for different fillings

Leeks, broccoli, sweet potatoes and chopped turkey meat.
Aubergines, red peppers, courgettes, onions and minced lamb.
Red onions, green peppers, canned or cooked haricot beans and celery.

CURRIED LENTILS

This versatile vegetable curry can be served just as it is with other curried dishes or it can be diluted with vegetable stock to make into a type of mulligatawny soup. Simply purée in a blender or rub through a sieve and serve garnished with a squeeze of lemon juice and some snipped chives. I sometimes make a much thicker version with less water to mix with cooked rice or to stuff into baked vegetables. Serve with Potato Dosas (see page 278)

Serves 4

4 tbsp extra virgin olive oil
1 onion, peeled and sliced

1 garlic clove, peeled and chopped

1 thick stick lemon grass

1 tbsp medium-strong curry powder

75g red or green split lentils

2 leeks, trimmed and chopped

1 red pepper, seeded and chopped

2 tbsp raisins

500ml water

1 tbsp tomato purée

freshly ground black pepper

For the garnish

juice of 1 lemon

2 tbsp freshly snipped chives

1 Heat the olive oil in a pan and gently fry the onions, garlic and lemon grass until golden in colour.

2 Add the curry powder and continue to fry for another minute or so.

3 Add all the remaining ingredients and bring to the boil. Cover with a lid and cook over a low to medium heat for 15–20 minutes. Check to see that the mixture is not boiling dry and stir from time to time. Alternatively, if the mixture is a little too thin for your purposes, thicken by boiling fast, uncovered, again stirring all the time.

4 Remove the lemon grass and sprinkle with lemon juice and chives to serve.

Healthy Highlights

With a wide variety of antioxidants in curry spices, such as the curcumin in turmeric, the softening of lentils in the presence of extra virgin olive oil maximises the absorption of the nutrients in the dish. Lentils contain fibre and also are a great source of folate, important for a healthy heart. Micronutrients, such as magnesium and iron, are also present in significant amounts, making lentils an excellent ingredient for the Olive Oil Diet.

LIGURIAN GREEN PIE

In Liguria, Italy, this pie would be made with *bietole* or wild greens gathered from the countryside, while a similar pie is made in Greece, again with wild greens or *horta*. However, the recipe works just as well with cultivated greens such as spinach, Swiss chard, beet leaves, kale or bok choy. Serve it on its own as a light lunch or with a salad.

Serves 4 (makes 500g pastry)

For the pastry
300g plain flour, plus extra for dusting
90ml extra virgin olive oil, plus extra for greasing
100ml water
1 egg yolk
For the filling
450g mixed greens
2 tbsp extra virgin olive oil, plus extra for greasing
1 onion, peeled and chopped
35g fresh parsley, roughly chopped
15g fresh basil or coriander, roughly chopped
3 eggs, lightly beaten
75g mature Pecorino cheese
freshly ground black pepper

1 Preheat the oven to 180°C/gas 4. Very lightly grease a non-stick, loose-based 20cm cake tin.

2 To make the pastry, sift the flour into a bowl. Beat together the olive oil and water and add the egg yolk. Pour the liquid mixture over the flour and mix to a smooth dough with your hands. Knead very lightly, if necessary, to bring it all together.

3 Cut the dough into two pieces, one weighing 300g and the other 200g. Roll out the larger piece on a floured surface and use it to line the prepared cake tin, leaving some of the pastry hanging over the edge. Roll out the remaining piece of pastry to make the top of the pie. Prick the base of the pie with a fork and chill while you make the filling.

4 To make the filling, steam the greens in very little water until soft and tender. Chop with a knife, making sure any stems are well cut up.

5 Meanwhile, heat the olive oil in pan and gently fry the onion until slightly softened.

6 Add the cooked greens and chopped herbs and continue cooking over a medium heat for 5 minutes. Transfer to a bowl and stir in the eggs and cheese. Season with pepper.

7 Spoon the filling mixture into the pastry case and moisten round the edge. Top with the lid, fold the pastry over and crimp round the top. Prick over the top with a fork and bake for 1 hour. You can cover the pie very lightly with a piece of foil to stop it browning too soon, but remove the foil half way through the cooking time.

8 Cut into wedges and serve hot.

SALADS AND COLD STARTERS

APPLE, FENNEL AND PUMPKIN SALAD

This is a really refreshing salad which can be served simply with lemon juice on a bed of rocket or as a more substantial salad mixed with Classic Mayonnaise (see page 179) and served with shelled crayfish or prawns. Prepare the fruit and vegetables quickly and toss them in the lemon juice straight away so that they don't discolour.

Serves 4

1 large apple, cored and finely chopped
3 tbsp lemon juice
½ small fennel bulb, trimmed and very finely chopped
6cm cucumber, finely chopped
4 tbsp Classic Mayonnaise (optional)
2 tbsp pumpkin seeds, toasted in a dry pan

1 Toss the apple in half the lemon juice, if you are adding mayonnaise later, or all the lemon juice if not. Add the fennel and cucumber and mix well. Add more lemon juice to taste or stir in the mayonnaise, if using.

2 Served sprinkled with the toasted pumpkin seeds.

GRAPEFRUIT AND AVOCADO
SALAD WITH FRESH HERBS

A quick and easy way of making breadcrumbs from fresh bread is to grate it on a coarse grater.

Serves 2

1 tbsp extra virgin olive oil

1 large slice wholemeal bread, made into crumbs

1 pink grapefruit, peeled

1 avocado, halved, stoned and peeled

3–4 sprigs fresh flatleaf parsley

1 small sprig fresh oregano

1 sprig fresh basil

For the dressing

4 tbsp extra virgin olive oil

1 tbsp red wine vinegar

freshly ground black pepper

1 Heat the olive oil in a hot frying pan and fry the breadcrumbs until crisp.

2 Segment the grapefruit and remove the membranes, reserving the juice. Arrange the segments of grapefruit in a circle on two serving plates.

3 Slice the avocado and place a slice between each grapefruit segment.

4 To make the dressing, mix the reserved grapefruit juice with the olive oil and vinegar, and season with pepper.

5 Pour the dressing over the salad. Roughly chop the herbs and mix with the fried breadcrumbs. Sprinkle them on top and serve at once.

Healthy Highlights

This is a powerhouse of nutrition. The drizzle of the olive oil dressing maximises the absorption of the vitamin E and phytonutrients, such as carotenoids, flavonoids and phytosterols from the avocado. The fat profile of avocados is excellent, being rich in monounsaturates. Avocado, like olive oil has been shown to improve blood glucose profile, so in combination with the grapefruit, this salad is excellent for those watching their weight. Grapefruit is also a great source of vitamin C. Heart-healthy parsley contains numerous antioxidants such as apigenin and luteolin, adding a wonderful garnish of antioxidants.

BABY LEAF AND PISTACHIO NUT SALAD

This salad goes well with others in a salad medley. Try serving it with Stuffed Chicory Spears with Eggs and Anchovies (see page 198) and Carrot and Orange Salad (see page 175). Alternatively serve it as a simple first course at the start of a more elaborate meal.

Serves 2

3–4 pieces sundried tomatoes
2 tbsp pistachio nuts
1 tbsp pine nuts
a handful watercress mixed with baby leaves
For the dressing
2 tbsp extra virgin olive oil
1 tsp sherry vinegar
freshly ground black pepper

1 If the sundried tomatoes are not packed in olive oil, soak in boiling water for 5–6 minutes, then drain. Cut the sundried tomatoes into thin strips and keep on one side.

2 Toast the pistachio nuts and pine nuts in a dry frying pan until lightly browned.

3 Arrange the baby leaves on two serving plates and sprinkle with the sundried tomatoes and toasted nuts.

4 Mix the dressing ingredients together, seasoning with pepper, and pour over the salad. Serve at once.

Suggestions

Add pumpkin seeds to the toasted nut mix.
Add mixed fresh herbs, such as basil leaves, to the baby leaf mix.

CARROT AND ORANGE SALAD

The combination of carrot and orange is a good one for salads. Do not make this salad too far in advance or, even with the dressing, the carrots will start to oxidize.

Serves 2

2 carrots, peeled and grated
1 small stick celery, very finely chopped
1 tablespoon raisins
a little grated orange zest
1 tablespoon extra virgin olive oil
1 tablespoon orange juice

Freshly ground black pepper

Freshly chopped tarragon, to garnish

1 Place the carrots and celery in a bowl and stir in the raisins and grated orange zest.

2 Mix the olive oil with the orange juice and black pepper and pour over the carrot mixture. Top with chopped tarragon and serve at once.

SPICED SUMMER SALAD

This salad is fun to make at the very beginning of the new potato season. It uses up all the very small potatoes that look pretty but get overcooked when put in with the others.

Serves 2

150g very small new potatoes

50g French beans, topped and tailed

25g fresh or frozen peas

1 well-flavoured tomato, cut into wedges

10–12 small Italian pickled onions in oil, drained and washed (optional)

1 tbsp chopped fresh coriander

For the dressing

2 tbsp olive oil

a few drops of oriental roast sesame oil or half and half olive oil and light sesame oil

1 tbsp sesame seeds

1cm fresh root ginger, peeled and grated

2 tbsp lemon juice

1 pinch cayenne pepper

1 Steam the new potatoes in a steamer for 5 minutes. Add the beans and peas and steam together for a further 5 minutes until just tender. Leave to cool.

2 Next make the dressing. Heat the oils in a pan and fry the seeds until lightly browned. Stir in the ginger, lemon juice and cayenne, then leave to cool.

3 Arrange the vegetables on plates with the tomato and onions. Sprinkle with coriander and pour on the cold dressing to serve.

WARM QUINOA SALAD

This is a great salad on which to serve fried fish fillets or chicken breasts which have been fried in olive oil. The recipe is just as good made with cooked couscous or bulgur so use whichever you have to hand. If you cannot find pickled lemons use half the amount of fresh lemons, chopped very finely indeed.

Serves 4

120g quinoa
300g water
75g fresh or frozen peas
4 fresh apricots, stoned and finely chopped
½ pickled lemon, seeds removed and chopped
2 spring onions, very finely chopped
4 tbsp extra virgin olive oil
1 tbsp lemon juice

1 Put the quinoa and water in a pan, bring to the boil, then reduce the heat and simmer for 15 minutes until all the liquid has been absorbed.

2 Meanwhile cook the peas in a little boiling water. When they are cooked, drain and add to the quinoa.

3 Mix the remaining salad ingredients into the quinoa and peas and toss with olive oil and lemon juice.

SICILIAN WINTER SALAD

The new season's fennel in Sicily is very different from the fennel that is usually found in northern Europe. It is very fresh and crunchy with a delicate aniseed flavour. It is wonderful in salads.

Serves 4

2 large fennel bulbs, trimmed and quartered
1 large handful rocket
1 orange, peeled and thinly sliced
16–20 small black olives, pitted
For the dressing
100ml extra virgin olive oil
juice of ½ lemon
1 pinch dried wild marjoram
salt and freshly ground black pepper

1 Place the fennel in a bowl of very cold water for 5 minutes. Drain and slice as finely as you can, preferably using a food processor or mandolin.

2 Arrange the rocket on a serving plate and top with slices of fennel and orange set in a pretty pattern. Dot with black olives.

3 Mix the olive oil with the lemon juice and dried herbs, then season with salt and pepper. Pour over the salad and serve.

AMERICAN APPLE AND CELERY SALAD

Originally known as Waldorf Salad in America from the hotel in which it was invented, this classic salad needs a good mayonnaise so do take the trouble to make you own if you can.

Serves 4

1 large green apple, with some of the peel removed
½ teaspoon lemon juice
4 sticks celery, sliced
8 walnut halves, coarsely chopped
4 tbsp Classic Mayonnaise (see below)

1 Core and finely chop the apple and mix with the lemon juice to prevent discolouring.

2 Add the celery and walnuts and mix well. Finally stir in the mayonnaise and serve at once.

CLASSIC MAYONNAISE

Mayonnaise is delicious made with extra virgin olive oil but it is best to choose an oil with a delicate flavour. I prefer to use an electric whisk rather than a food processor as I feel I am more in control. However, if you are in a hurry and want to use the processor, use the pulse button rather than putting the machine on full power all the time.

Makes 300ml

2 egg yolks
1 pinch salt

½ teaspoon dry mustard (optional)

1 tbsp white wine vinegar or lemon juice

300ml extra virgin olive oil

freshly ground black pepper

1 tbsp boiling water

1 Place the egg yolks in a large bowl and whisk for about 2 minutes. Add the salt, mustard, if using, and the vinegar or lemon juice and whisk again.

2 Keep whisking and very slowly add the oil almost drop by drop. When half the oil has been absorbed you can start adding the remainder by the tablespoonful.

3 Finally season with black pepper and add the boiling water to stabilise the mayonnaise.

4 Cover and store in the fridge. Use within a week.

HERRING AND BEETROOT SALAD

This salad makes an excellent snack or first course without the eggs. Add the eggs and serve with Sprouted Soda Bread (see page 266) for a more substantial meal. Alternatively, serve in a salad medley with two or three other salads.

Serves 4

2–3 rollmop herrings, depending on size

2 cooked beetroot, peeled and cubed

1 pickled cucumber, finely chopped

1 large apple, cored and cubed

3 tbsp extra virgin olive oil

1 tbsp lemon juice

freshly ground black pepper

2 hard-boiled eggs, sliced (optional)

1 Cut the rollmops into bite-sized pieces and place in a large bowl with the beetroot, pickled cucumber and apple.

2 Beat the olive oil and lemon juice with the pepper and pour over the salad ingredients.

3 Toss everything well together. Serve on its own or garnished with sliced hard-boiled eggs, if you like.

WARM SALAD OF MIXED GRILLED VEGETABLES

Serve this colourful salad as a side dish for grilled chicken or burgers in a bun. Alternatively, leave to cool a little and top with slices of grilled goat's cheese. Serve with Cheese Muffins (see page 268).

Serves 4

1 medium-sized aubergine

2 small courgettes

1 red pepper

4 tbsp extra virgin olive oil

1 handful mixed salad leaves

For the dressing

4 tbsp extra virgin olive oil

1 tbsp sherry vinegar

1 Cut the aubergine into slices and then into sticks. Do the same with the courgettes. Deseed the pepper and cut into strips. Preheat the grill.

2 Line a grill pan with foil and arrange the vegetable strips in a single layer on the foil. Drizzle with the olive oil.

3 Place under a hot grill for 5 minutes. Toss or stir the vegetables from time to time so that they cook evenly on all sides.

4 Arrange the salad leaves on serving plates. Whisk together the dressing ingredients.

5 Toss the vegetables with a fork and spread out again on the foil. Cook for a further 3–5 minutes until the vegetables are lightly browned but still have a touch of crunchiness to them.

6 Spoon the vegetables over the prepared salad, drizzle with the dressing and serve at once.

Suggestions

Choose red wine, balsamic or herb-flavoured vinegar instead of red wine vinegar.

Substitute a fennel bulb, thinly sliced and cut into sticks, in place of the courgettes or peppers.

FIG AND BLACK OLIVE TAPENADE WITH ROCKET SALAD

This variation on the usual black olive tapenade makes a great spread for fried bread croûtons. Use it to make canapés or serve as a light lunch or first course on a rocket salad. You can, of course, use any kind of olive tapenade or anchoiade for this dish.

Serves 4 (makes 12 canapés)

4 ready-to-eat dried figs, stems trimmed, quartered
250ml water
100g pitted Kalamata olives
½ tsp fennel seeds, crushed
2 tsp grated lemon zest
½ tsp freshly ground black pepper
5 tbsp extra virgin olive oil
4 rounds French bread
For the rocket salad
2 tbsp pumpkin seeds
6 Brazil nuts, chopped
1 large handful rocket
4 sundried tomato halves in olive oil, sliced into thin strips

1 Place the figs and in a small saucepan. Bring to the boil. Cover and cook over low heat until almost all of the liquid has been absorbed, about 20 minutes. Cool slightly.

2 Combine the figs, olives, fennel seeds, lemon zest and black pepper in a food processor. Process until puréed, stopping to scrape the sides of the container down once or twice. With the motor running, slowly add 2 tablespoons olive oil.

3 Transfer the mixture to a container or bowl, cover and refrigerate until ready to use.

4 Meanwhile, brush the rounds of French bread with 1 tablespoon olive oil and fry in a dry frying pan until crisp and golden.

5 Spread with the black olive and fig tapenade mixture.

6 To make the salad, toast the pumpkin seeds and chopped Brazil nuts in a dry frying pan until lightly browned.

7 Arrange the rocket on serving plates and place a tapenade croûte in the centre of each plate. Place the sundried tomato strips around the outside and sprinkle with the seeds and nuts. Finally, drizzle with the rest of the olive oil to serve.

Healthy Highlight

Not only does this recipe include the health benefits of olives and olive oil, but the addition of figs, fennel seeds and lemon zest brings a medley of flavours without the need for salt. Figs are a good source of fibre and potassium which helps to reduce blood pressure. Lemon will reduce the glycaemic load of the combination.

CAULIFLOWER AND RED PEPPER SALAD

This is a colourful and tasty salad to serve in a salad medley or as an accompaniment to a nut roast.

Serves 2

1 baby cauliflower
1 large red pepper, seeded and cut into quarters
4 sprigs fresh tarragon
4 large sprigs fresh flatleaf parsley

20 black olives, pitted and quartered
For the dressing
2 tbsp extra virgin olive oil
1 tsp red wine vinegar
freshly ground black pepper

1 Steam the cauliflower for 4–5 minutes – it should still have some bite to it. Leave to cool and break into florets.

2 Grill the pepper until the skin browns and blisters. Leave to stand for 5 minutes, then peel off the skin. Cut into strips.

3 Chop 1 large sprig of tarragon and mix with the dressing ingredients. Leave to stand until required.

4 Arrange the parsley on serving plates. Place the pepper strips on top of the parsley. Dot with cauliflower florets and sprinkle with olives.

5 Spoon the dressing over the top and finish with the remaining sprigs of tarragon. Serve at once.

Suggestions

Add ½ crushed garlic clove to the dressing.
Sprinkle the salad with chopped Brazil nuts or hazelnuts.

THREE-FRUIT SALAD

Balsamic vinegar of Modena can be very good but it can also be very bad. Check the label for the ingredients. These should simply be cooked grape must and aged wine vinegar, preferably listed in that order. Do not buy those with caramel, preservatives or other additives. Serve this dish as a savoury first course or light lunch dish.

Serves 4

1 kiwi fruit, peeled and sliced

1 Sharon fruit, sliced

1 tomato, sliced

1 handful mixed salad leaves

1 tbsp Brazil nuts, toasted in a dry pan, then chopped

1 small goat's cheese log, thinly sliced

1 tbsp black olives

a few sprigs fresh parsley or basil

For the dressing

3 tbsp extra virgin olive oil

1 tsp good quality balsamic vinegar of Modena

freshly ground black pepper

1 Arrange slices of the fruits in an overlapping rosette on each plate. Place a little mixed leaves adjacent to it and fill in the space with slices of goat's cheese. Place black olives at each junction to make an attractive arrangement and dot with parsley or basil.

2 Mix together the dressing ingredients, seasoning with pepper to taste, and sprinkle all over, but particularly on the fruit and leaves.

Healthy Highlights

The Olive Oil Diet is rich in fruit as well as vegetables, and here is a great way to celebrate the vitamins, potassium, minerals and fibre of fruit in a savoury dish. Combining with nuts adds good fats and other trace minerals, such as selenium, important for enzymic processes in the body. Balsamic vinegar has been the subject of research suggesting it may have a beneficial effect on blood pressure and cholesterol oxidation as well as glycaemic load.

POTATO SALAD WITH EGG AND CAPER SAUCE

Egg and caper sauce also goes well with green salads and with cold sliced chicken. You can use old or new potatoes for the salad.

Serves 4

600g potatoes, peeled
freshly ground black pepper
For the egg and caper sauce
1 egg
3 tbsp finely chopped fresh parsley
50g capers, roughly chopped
a little chopped garlic
100ml extra virgin olive oil

1 Cook the potatoes in boiling water until tender. Drain and season with black pepper. Leave to cool.

2 Meanwhile, hard-boil the egg, then chop it finely. Leave to cool.

3 Mix the hard-boiled egg with the parsley, capers and chopped garlic. Stir into the olive oil.

4 Arrange the potatoes in a bowl and pour on the sauce to serve.

SPICED TABBOULEH SALAD

This Middle Eastern speciality makes a refreshing accompaniment to almost any grilled foods.

Serves 4

50g bulgur
6 tbsp chopped fresh parsley
½ small red pepper, seeded and finely chopped
4 tbsp extra virgin olive oil
1 tbsp lemon juice
¼ tsp ground cinnamon
¼ tsp ground coriander
freshly ground black pepper
For the garnish
chopped walnuts
pomegranate seeds

1 Place the bulgur in a bowl and cover with boiling water. Leave to stand for 30 minutes.

2 Drain very well, squeezing out all the water with your fingers. Leave to cool.

3 Just before serving, mix the bulgur with all the remaining ingredients and top with chopped walnuts and pomegranate seeds.

Healthy Highlights

This dish is based on bulgur, a wholegrain with plenty of fibre as well as locked-in minerals. This traditional wheat which has been eaten in the Middle East for centuries was recently associated with lower levels of chemicals in the blood, which are markers for inflammation. Walnuts are a great source of heart-healthy fats and vitamins. Pomegranate seeds are packed with vitamins C and K and have plenty of polyphenol antioxidants as well.

RAVIOLI AND BROCCOLI SALAD

This is a stunning salad which looks fantastic on a cold buffet. It can also be served as a meal in its own right. It needs a good punchy oil so try using an extra virgin olive oil from Central Italy or from California.

Serves 4

20g dried porcini mushrooms
boiling water
200g broccoli florets
100ml Californian or Italian extra virgin olive oil
1 garlic clove, peeled and crushed
1 tsp soy sauce
25ml red wine vinegar
½ tsp dried tarragon
1 pinch dry mustard
250g small ravioli filled with ricotta cheese
4–5 spring onions or a small bunch chives, finely chopped
2 tbsp freshly grated Parmesan cheese
salt and freshly ground black pepper

1 Just cover the dried mushrooms with boiling water and leave to stand for 30 minutes.

2 Steam the broccoli florets until *al dente*, then refresh in cold water. Cut them into smaller pieces if very large.

3 Strain the mushrooms, keeping the liquid for another dish, and chop finely.

4 Heat 1 tablespoon olive oil and gently fry the mushrooms and garlic for 5 minutes.

5 Add the soy sauce and boil until the liquid has reduced. Keep on one side with the broccoli.

6 Cook the ravioli in boiling salted water with a splash of olive oil for 6–8 minutes until just tender. Drain, rinse under cold water and drain again, then leave to cool.

7 Next make the dressing by mixing the vinegar, tarragon and the remaining olive oil. Season with salt and pepper.

8 To put the salad together, place the broccoli, the mushroom and garlic mixture and the ravioli in a bowl and toss gently with the spring onions or chives and the dressing. Sprinkle with a little Parmesan cheese and serve.

FISH TARTAR

Any kind of oily fish, such as tuna or salmon, is suitable for this classy first course but it needs to be as fresh as possible. Prepare the dish the day before and store in the fridge overnight. Serve on crostini or use to make interesting canapés on small squares of fried bread.

Serves 4 (makes 12 canapés)

300g fresh salmon, skinned and pin boned
4 spring onions, finely chopped
2 tbsp drained capers, chopped

2 tbsp chopped fresh mint

2 tbsp extra virgin olive oil

grated rind and juice of ½ large lemon

1 pinch salt, to taste

freshly ground black pepper

To serve

a few handfuls rocket

extra virgin olive oil

3 slices bread

1 Chop the salmon finely.

2 Combine with all the other ingredients, seasoning with salt and pepper to taste, and refrigerate overnight.

3 Serve with a little rocket salad drizzled with olive oil. Or spread onto bread fried in olive oil and cut each round into four pieces.

ESCALIVADA

This Spanish cooked vegetable salad makes a good first course but it can also be served as part of a Spanish tapas spread. It is best made in advance and left to stand for a while before serving. That gives the flavours time to mingle with the oil to make the taste even better. It's great served with Oatcakes (see page 275).

Serves 4

1 aubergine

2 large red peppers

5–6 tbsp extra virgin olive oil

freshly ground black pepper

1 Preheat the oven to 190°C/gas 5.

2 Place the aubergine and peppers on a baking tray and cook in the oven for about 20–30 minutes until they are well browned. Leave to cool and then peel.

3 Cut the aubergines into long strips and the peppers into shorter ones.

4 Arrange a row of aubergine strips on a serving plate and interlace the red pepper strips with the aubergine to give a lattice effect.

5 Spoon on the olive oil and grind the black pepper over the top.

6 Leave to stand until required.

CHICKEN SALSA VERDE WITH NEW POTATOES

The *salsa verde* can be made in advance and kept in the fridge for two or three days. It is a very versatile sauce for all kinds of cold meats. It also makes an excellent dipping sauce for globe artichokes.

Serves 4

500g new potatoes
1 small cold cooked chicken
1 large handful watercress
For the salsa verde
1 egg
5–6 anchovy fillets, chopped
3 tbsp chopped fresh parsley
3 tbsp finely chopped cornichons or small gherkins
2 tbsp drained capers, chopped
1 garlic clove, peeled and crushed
juice of 1 lemon

6 tbsp extra virgin olive oil
freshly ground black pepper

1 Steam the potatoes until tender. Use hot or cold, as you prefer.

2 Hard-boil the egg for the salsa, leave to cool, then chop.

3 Strip the meat from the chicken and slice.

4 Make the salsa by mixing the hard-boiled egg, anchovies, parsley, cornichons, capers and garlic in a bowl. Stir in the lemon juice, olive oil and black pepper.

5 To serve, arrange the chicken and new potatoes on serving plates. Spoon the *salsa verde* over the top and serve with a little watercress on the side.

TUNA AND GREEN BEAN SALAD

The best bean sprouts to use in this main-course salad are the English-style bean shoots which are much shorter than the usual Chinese mung bean sprouts. Serve with Greek yogurt on the side and slices of Sprouted Soda Bread (see page 266).

Serves 4

1 x 160g can tuna steaks
75g cooked green beans, cut into short pieces
50g English bean sprouts or sprouted chickpeas
2 tbsp finely chopped fresh parsley
1 tbsp finely chopped red onion
3 small gherkins, finely chopped (optional)
1 tbsp lemon juice
1 tbsp olive oil
freshly ground black pepper

To serve

Greek yogurt

Sprouted Soda Bread (see page 262)

1 Drain and flake the tuna and place in a mixing bowl. Add all the remaining ingredients and toss carefully together. Try not to break up the tuna too much. You may need to add more olive oil if the tuna was not packed in oil.

2 Serve with Greek yogurt and soda bread.

Healthy Highlights

This is a typical fusion of excellent nutrition so often seen with combining the ingredients of the Olive Oil Diet. Olive oil adds to the moisture of the meal, combining its uniquely powerful tyrosol anti-oxidants with the Omega-3 fats of the tuna and the fibre and B vitamins in the green beans. Red onions pack a powerful punch,with the outer layers containing extraordinarily high levels of polyphenol antioxidants including anthocyanins and quercetin.

PECORINO SALAD WITH FRUIT AND OLIVES

This really is an all-the-year-round salad. Choose fruit in season and any kind of good green olives. Serve as a first course or as a good lunchtime snack with plenty of wholemeal bread.

Serves 4

3 tender lettuce hearts, washed and drained

1 pink grapefruit, peeled and segmented

1 sweet apple, cored and diced

200g Pecorino cheese, crumbled or diced

100g green table olives, pitted

6cm cucumber, diced

2 small spring onions, finely chopped

juice of 1 lemon

5 tbsp extra virgin olive oil

1 Tear the lettuce leaves into pieces by hand and use to line a salad bowl.

2 Cut the grapefruit segments into small pieces and mix with the apple, cheese, olives, cucumber and spring onions. Spoon this mixture onto the lettuce leaves.

3 Beat the lemon juice with olive oil to taste and pour over the salad. Toss gently and serve at once.

CHICKEN AND SPROUTED CHICKPEA SALAD

Serve this lovely crunchy salad with a Crisp Rosemary Flatbread (see page 277).

Serves 4

1 medium-sized fennel bulb, trimmed and thinly sliced

225g cooked chicken meat, roughly chopped

225g seedless grapes, cut in half

100g sprouted chickpeas

4 sprigs fresh mint, roughly chopped

4–5 tbsp Classic Mayonnaise (see page 179)

To serve

mixed salad leaves

Crisp Rosemary Flatbread

1 Steam the fennel for about 5–6 minutes to soften just a little. Leave to cool while you make the flatbread.

2 Chop the steamed fennel and mix with all the other ingredients.

3 Serve on a bed of mixed salad leaves with the hot flatbread.

Healthy Highlights

Chickpeas are high in fibre and many minerals, whilst fennel contains an interesting antioxidant called anethole, giving its typical aniseed flavour and which has strong anti-inflammatory properties. Rosemary contains aspirin-like anti-inflammatory salicylates as well as the anti-oxidant rosemarinic acid, also present in mint. Serve with a drizzle of extra virgin olive oil, as always.

STUFFED ROMANO PEPPERS WITH CHICORY AND CELERY SALAD

This salad looks as good as it tastes. If Romano peppers are not available, use small to medium-sized red peppers instead.

Serves 4

4 red peppers
For the stuffing
300g Greek yogurt
50g sprouted chickpeas, roughly chopped
50g cashew nuts, finely chopped
2 tbsp finely chopped fresh dill
1 tbsp sunflower seeds

1 tbsp finely chopped red onion

For the chicory and celery salad

3–4 small heads chicory, sliced

2–3 sticks celery, sliced

1 small orange, peeled and chopped

2 tbsp extra virgin olive oil

1 tsp lemon juice

1 Cut the tops off the peppers and scoop out all the seeds. Keep on one side.

2 Mix the Greek yogurt with all the other stuffing ingredients to form a stiff paste. Spoon this mixture into the red peppers and refrigerate for 1 hour.

3 When you are ready to serve, toss the salad ingredients together in a bowl.

4 Cut the stuffed peppers into rings and serve with the salad on the side.

Suggestion

If time is short, try stuffing the peppers with ready-made houmous or guacamole.

STUFFED CHICORY SPEARS WITH EGGS AND ANCHOVIES

Serve this delicious dish as a first course or double the quantities and serve as a light meal with Sprouted Soda Bread (see page 266). Choose anchovies which have been packed in olive oil.

Serves 4

4 eggs

2 tbsp Classic Mayonnaise (see page 179)

10 small cherry tomatoes, finely chopped

2 tbsp chopped fresh coriander

3–4 heads Belgian endive or chicory

8 anchovy fillets

extra virgin olive oil

1 Hard-boil the eggs, then roughly chop. Add the mayonnaise and mash with a fork. Stir in the tomatoes and coriander and keep on one side.

2 Peel off 16 large spears from the endive, keeping the small centre leaves for another salad.

3 Arrange four spears on each plate. Spoon the egg and tomato mixture down the centre of each spear and top with an anchovy fillet.

4 Serve drizzled with plenty of olive oil.

Suggestion

Omit the anchovies for a vegetarian menu.

SEAFOOD SALPICON SALAD

This really refreshing salad comes from Extremadura in western Spain and often forms part of a tapas meal. However, it also makes a great lunch dish in its own right and in smaller quantities can be served as a first course.

Serves 4

400g frozen cooked mixed seafood, including prawns, calamari and
   mussels
1 large apple, cored and very finely chopped
1 large tomato, very finely chopped
1 green pepper, seeded and very finely chopped
1 small onion, peeled and very finely chopped
4 tbsp extra virgin olive oil
1 tbsp white wine vinegar
1 bunch watercress

1 Thaw and drain the seafood and place in a serving dish or on individual plates.
2 Mix all the remaining ingredients in a bowl and spoon over the seafood just before serving.
3 Dot with sprigs of watercress to serve.

CHEF'S SHREDDED SALAD

This is a versatile salad as you can add any vegetables, cheese or meat which you happen to have in the fridge such as leftover roasts and even cooked vegetables such as peas or broccoli.

Serves 4

½ head Chinese leaves, shredded

½ green pepper, seeded and cut into thin strips

1 carrot, peeled and cut into thin strips

½ small celeriac, peeled and cut into thin strips

1 handful Chinese beansprouts

150g cooked chicken, shredded

100g semi-soft cheese such as Gouda or tilsit, cut into strips

Classic Mayonnaise (see page 179)

1 Place all the vegetables in a bowl and add the Chinese beansprouts. Add the chicken and cheese to the bowl.

2 Carefully stir in the mayonnaise, taking care not to break the strips of meat or vegetables.

3 For the best results, chill for 15 minutes before serving, but do not chill for too long or the mixture will thicken.

SOUPS AND HOT STARTERS

CHICKPEA BROTH WITH CORIANDER

The unusual flavour of this very quick soup depends upon the whole dried coriander seeds. Resist the temptation to add fresh coriander as a garnish. The fresh herb will take over completely. To turn the broth into a main meal, serve with fried croûtons topped with grated mature Pecorino cheese.

Serves 4

50ml extra virgin olive oil
1 tbsp whole coriander seeds
2 small onions, peeled and sliced
100g small button mushrooms
100g cooked or canned, drained chickpeas
1 tsp dried oregano
1 bay leaf
300ml white wine
400ml tomato juice
1 small fresh red chilli pepper
freshly ground black pepper

1 Heat the olive oil and fry the whole coriander seeds for 30 seconds.

2 Add the onions and continue to fry gently for another 2–3 minutes.

3 Add all the remaining ingredients and bring to the boil. Cook, uncovered, for 18–20 minutes to concentrate the flavour.

ROQUEFORT AND CELERIAC SOUP

Blue cheeses go very well with a variety of vegetables to make excellent soups. Celeriac gives a distinctive but delicate flavour to this soup. If you do not want to use cream, use yogurt with a little potato flour creamed into to it to stop the yogurt from curdling.

Serves 4

3 tbsp extra virgin olive oil
2 onions, peeled and sliced
450g celeriac, peeled and diced
1 carrot, peeled and diced
750ml chicken or vegetable stock
150ml single cream
125g Roquefort cheese, crumbled
freshly ground black pepper

1 Heat the olive oil in a pan and gently fry the onions, celeriac and carrot for 3–4 minutes to bring out the flavours.

2 Add the stock, season with pepper and bring to the boil. Cover and simmer for 20 minutes.

3 Purée in a blender, return to the saucepan and add the cream and cheese. Carefully reheat, stirring all the time, until the cheese melts. Serve at once.

Suggestions

Here are some other combinations that work well:
Beenleigh Blue cheese with broccoli
Lanark Blue cheese with cauliflower

MARROW AND PEPPER SOUP WITH GARLIC BREAD

Marrows are great stuffed with onions and tomato as a vegetable dish or cubed and served with a dill cream sauce, but they also make excellent soups. You can use any colour of sweet pepper you like for this soup.

Serves 4–6 as a main course

600g marrow, peeled, seeded and chopped
1 courgette, chopped
1 red pepper, seeded and chopped
1 green pepper, seeded and chopped
50ml extra virgin olive oil
1 small bunch chives, 2 or 3 spring onions or a shallot
2 sprigs fresh basil (optional)
450ml water
freshly ground black pepper
For the garlic bread
50ml extra virgin olive oil
2–3 garlic cloves, peeled and crushed
1 long stick French bread

1 Heat the olive oil in a pan, add the vegetables and fry over a gentle heat for about 5 minutes until beginning to soften.

2 Add all the remaining ingredients and bring to the boil. Cover and simmer for 30 minutes until all the vegetables are tender.

3 Meanwhile, to make the garlic bread, preheat the oven to 200°C/gas 6.

4 Heat the olive oil in a small saucepan and cook the garlic for a few minutes until it just begins to turn golden in colour. Remove from the heat immediately.

5 Cut the French loaf in half, then cut each piece in half lengthways. Brush the bread all over with the garlic olive oil and put the two sides back together again to make two lengths of bread.

6 Wrap in foil and bake for about 15 minutes until crisp.

7 When the soup is ready, purée in a blender or rub through a sieve, then return to the pan and reheat gently before serving with the garlic bread.

CELERY AND TOMATO SOUP WITH PARSLEY

Turn this soup into a more substantial dish by topping with a slice of wholegrain bread fried in olive oil and topped with grated Pecorino cheese.

Serves 4

1 small head celery, sliced
250g tomatoes, roughly chopped
150g carrots, peeled and chopped
1 bay leaf
freshly grated nutmeg
plenty of freshly ground black pepper
500ml water
3 tablespoons extra virgin olive oil, plus extra for serving

40g chopped fresh parsley
To serve
cheese croûtons (optional)

1 Place the celery, tomatoes and carrots in a saucepan and add the bay leaf, nutmeg and black pepper. Pour on the water and olive oil and bring to the boil.
2 Cover with a lid, reduce the heat and simmer for 45 minutes.
3 Purée in a blender or rub through a sieve, then return to the heat. Stir in the chopped parsley just before serving and top with large cheese croûtons, if using.
4 Serve more olive oil on the side to swirl into the soup.

Healthy Highlights

From the apigenin in celery, to the lycopenes in tomatoes, the carotenoids in carrots and the polyphenols in extra virgin olive oil, this recipe provides a wonderful medley of natural antioxidants.

SOUPE AU PISTOU

The lovely fresh vegetables in this soup from the south of France do not need too much cooking. For the best effect, keep them crunchy.

Serves 4

4 tbsp extra virgin olive oil
1 large onion, peeled and chopped
2 leeks, trimmed and cut into rounds

2 carrots, peeled and diced

1 large potato, peeled and diced

50g macaroni

3 tomatoes, peeled and chopped

225g courgettes, sliced

75g French beans, cut into lengths

1 handful fresh or frozen peas

½ x 415g can cannellini beans, drained

For the pistou

2–3 garlic cloves, peeled and chopped

1 bunch fresh basil

50g Parmesan cheese, freshly grated

3–4 tbsp olive oil

freshly ground black pepper

1 Heat the olive oil in a saucepan and gently fry the onion and leeks until slightly softened.

2 Add the carrots and potato and toss in the oil. Cover with water and bring to the boil. Simmer for 15 minutes.

3 Add the macaroni and continue simmering for 10 minutes.

4 Add all the remaining soup ingredients and simmer for another 5 minutes.

5 Meanwhile, make the *pistou* by processing the garlic with the basil in a blender. Take care not to over-process the herbs.

6 Add half the Parmesan cheese and the oil to the soup and season with black pepper. Serve the soup in bowls garnished with the remaining Parmesan and with the *pistou* in a separate bowl on the side for diners to help themselves.

LENTIL AND CARROT SOUP WITH WATERCRESS SALSA

Serve this warming winter soup with Crispy Potato Cakes (see page 278). You can easily make both within an hour.

Serves 4

1 tbsp extra virgin olive oil
1 onion, peeled and sliced
150g carrots, peeled and chopped
50g red or green split lentils
700ml water
½ tsp dried thyme or 2 sprigs fresh thyme
1 bay leaf
freshly ground black pepper
For the watercress salsa
1 bunch watercress
4 large sprigs fresh parsley
100ml extra virgin olive oil

1 Heat the olive oil in a pan and gently fry the onion until beginning to turn gold.

2 Add the carrots, lentils, water, herbs and pepper and bring to the boil. Reduce the heat, cover with a lid and simmer for 30 minutes.

3 Remove the sprig of thyme and the bay leaf. Purée the soup in a blender or rub through a sieve, then return the soup to the pan and reheat gently.

4 Meanwhile, make the salsa by blending the watercress, parsley and oil in a blender or food processor. Take care not to over-process or the herbs will be too fine and tasty gritty.

5 Spoon the soup into bowls and serve with the salsa on the side.

PORTUGUESE-STYLE DRY SOUP WITH
ROMANESCO AND PEPPERS

Dry soups are made with bread and in some ways are more like a hotpot than a soup. Instead of ladling the soup over the bread in the Italian tradition, the bread is placed over the soup and baked to give a deliciously crunchy topping. Use boned chicken for a faster result. Romanesco is sometimes labelled as broccoletti.

Serves 4

6 tbsp extra virgin olive oil
2 large chicken leg joints, trimmed and skinned
450ml chicken stock
1 romanesco head, trimmed and cut into chunky florets
1 onion, peeled, cut into thick rings and coarsely chopped
2 red peppers, seeded and coarsely chopped
2–3 sprigs fresh lemon thyme
4 slices bread
freshly ground black pepper

1 Preheat the oven to 200°C/gas 6.

2 Place 3 tablespoons olive oil in a heavy-based ovenproof saucepan and add the chicken joints. Fry quickly until they are lightly browned all over.

3 Pour on the stock and season with black pepper. Bring the mixture to the boil, then cover with a lid, reduce the heat and simmer for 15–20 minutes until the chicken is cooked through.

4 Remove the chicken from the pan and keep on one side.

5 Add the romanesco, onion, peppers and thyme to the stock pan. Cover again and simmer for a further 10 minutes.

6 Meanwhile, remove the chicken meat from the bones and slice into strips. Return to the pan with the vegetables and sprigs of thyme and mix together.

7 Arrange the slices of bread on the top of soup, pressing it down to take up a little of the juices. Drizzle the remaining olive oil over the top and place in the preheated oven.

8 Bake for 10 minutes until the bread is golden.

Suggestions

Use kale, cauliflower or broccoli in place of romanesco.

THICK BEAN AND CABBAGE SOUP

Based loosely on Italian *ribollita*, this hearty soup makes a great winter meal served with hunks of homemade Sprouted Soda Bread (see page 266). If you want to try something a little more authentic, it is now possible to get Tuscan black cabbage outside Italy. This cabbage will take longer to cook than Savoy cabbage.

Serves 4–6

75g white haricot or cannellini beans, soaked in cold water overnight
    and drained
1.8 litres vegetable stock
1 tbsp extra virgin olive oil
1 onion, peeled and finely chopped
1 garlic clove, peeled and finely chopped
1 small sprig fresh rosemary

1 fresh bay leaf

2 sticks celery, thinly sliced

1 carrot, peeled and finely diced

1 tablespoon tomato purée

1 small to medium Savoy cabbage, shredded

freshly ground black pepper

1 Place the beans in a pan with 725ml of the stock, bring to the boil, then cover with a lid and simmer gently for about 1 hour until the beans are tender. If the beans are old this could take a bit longer. Remove half of the beans and keep on one side.

2 Heat the oil in a frying pan and gently fry the onion, garlic, rosemary, bay leaf, celery and carrot for 10 minutes until soft but not brown. Remove the rosemary and bay leaf. Add to the soup pan with the remaining stock, the tomato purée and cabbage and season with pepper. Return to the boil and simmer for 15 minutes.

3 Purée the reserved beans or rub through a sieve, then add to the soup. Check and adjust the seasoning to taste and cook for further 10 minutes.

PRAWNS SAN LUCAR

Southern Spain is home to this rather special dish which uses mouth-watering fried croûtons to help cut the cost of the prawns. Serve as a first course or as a lunch dish.

Serves 4

228g can tomatoes

1 bunch spring onions, finely chopped

½ tsp dried oregano

1 pinch fennel seed or herb

salt and freshly ground black pepper

75ml extra virgin olive oil

4 slices white bread

250g peeled prawns

juice of ½ lemon

chopped fresh parsley

1 Empty the can of tomatoes into a pan and chop. Add the spring onions, herbs and seasonings and bring to the boil. Cover with a lid and simmer for 15–20 minutes.

2 Meanwhile heat the olive oil and fry the bread until crisp and golden on each side. Drain on kitchen paper and cut into cubes.

3 Add the prawns to the tomato mixture and heat through (or cook until pink, if fresh). Either way the prawns should not be cooked for too long or they will go hard.

4 Add the bread cubes, toss and serve immediately sprinkled with lemon juice and parsley, with some more olive oil on the side, as always.

Healthy Highlights

All the natural ingredients in this healthy recipe have their own unique health profiles. However, it is the prawns which are the main star of the dish. Prawns are a great source of Omega-3s and contain the minerals selenium and copper, which are involved in enzyme processes in the body. Prawns are particularly rich in a carotenoid compound called axtasanthin which is a powerful antioxidant.

BAKED FETA CHEESE WITH TOMATOES

This is such a quick and easy dish to make that it is a great standby for a late supper or light lunch but it is also very good served as part of a Greek meze. You can make individual parcels for each diner, if you prefer.

Serves 4

400g sheep's milk feta cheese
1 large beef tomato, very finely sliced
2 tbsp dried oregano
3–4 tbsp extra virgin olive oil
freshly ground black pepper

1 Preheat the oven to 190°C/gas 4.

2 Place the cheese on a large square of kitchen foil and top with the sliced tomatoes and oregano. Finish with olive oil and black pepper, then wrap up into a loose closed parcel.

3 Place on a baking tray and bake for 8–10 minutes. Open the parcel and serve from the foil.

Suggestion

Add some pitted green or black olives to the parcel.

STUFFED AND GRILLED LITTLE GEM LETTUCES

This recipe uses the heart of the gem lettuce, so if the lettuces are quite large, remove the outer leaves and use in a mixed salad. This dish makes an excellent first course.

Serves 4

6 little gem lettuces, cut in half
extra virgin olive oil
For the stuffing
2 tbsp drained capers
3 tbsp raisins or sultanas
3 tbsp pine nuts, toasted in a dry pan
16 black olives, pitted and quartered
2–3 small spring onions, finely chopped
½ tsp dried oregano or 1 small sprig fresh oregano
freshly ground black pepper

1 Place the capers and raisins or sultanas in a cup and cover with water. Leave to stand for 10 minutes.

2 Drain, dry and chop with the pine nuts and olives.

3 Stir in the spring onions and mix with 3 tablespoons of olive oil, plenty of black pepper and a little oregano.

4 Place the gem lettuces cut-side down on a foil-lined tray and drizzle with olive oil. Grill for 2–3 minutes until very lightly charred at the edges. Turn them over, drizzle more oil on the flat surfaces and grill again for about 2 minutes to soften the centres.

5 Spread with the stuffing mixture and grill for a final 2–3 minutes.

6 Serve at once, finished with more olive oil.

BROCCOLI WITH RED PEPPERS AND HAZELNUTS

Serve this dish on its own as a great starter or serve in a mixed medley of vegetable dishes. Alternatively sprinkle with crumbled feta cheese and serve with chunky wholemeal rolls for a more substantial dish.

Serves 4

2 small to medium-size red peppers, seeded and quartered
60ml extra virgin olive oil
1 large head broccoli, divided into florets
2 tbsp chopped hazelnuts, toasted in a dry pan

1 Put the pepper in a shallow pan and drizzle with the olive oil. Cover with a lid and place on a medium heat. As soon as the oil starts to sizzle, reduce the heat and cook over a low heat for about 30 minutes until tender. Cut into strips and leave in the pan juices.

2 Meanwhile steam the broccoli in a steamer for about 10 minutes until just tender.

3 Transfer the broccoli to a serving dish and top with the pepper strips and their juices.

4 Finish by sprinkling on the toasted nuts.

Healthy Highlights

The sulphur-containing compounds in broccoli are well known for their healthy properties. Hazelnuts were one of the nuts used in the Predimed Study which demonstrated the benefits of a nut and extra virgin olive oil supplemented Mediterranean Diet.

GRILLED PRAWNS WITH CORIANDER 'MOJO'

El mojo is a kind of dressing or sauce which is very popular in the Canary Islands. It is always made with extra virgin olive oil and it may simply be spicy or it may be very hot with chilli or paprika. This version is a green mojo made with coriander leaves and fresh green peppers, such as *padron*, which are not spicy.

Serves 4

1 bunch fresh coriander, roughly chopped
3 garlic cloves, peeled and chopped
2 green peppers, seeded and chopped
1 tsp ground cumin
1 tsp coarse sea salt
150ml Spanish or Portuguese extra virgin olive oil
50ml white wine vinegar
1kg unpeeled raw prawns

1 Start by making the mojo. Place the coriander, garlic, peppers, cumin and salt in a mortar and crush it all very well together, or blend in a blender or processor.

2 Then add the olive oil slowly, whisking or processing all the time. Finally add the vinegar and leave to stand until required.

3 Grill the prawns under a hot grill until pink, then serve at once.

4 Hand round the mojo sauce to spoon on the prawns once they are peeled.

STUFFED MUSHROOMS WITH CASHEWS AND ROQUEFORT

This mushroom dish makes a great first course and is quite quick to prepare.

Serves 2

4 large Portobello or field mushrooms
125ml extra virgin olive oil
1 large onion, peeled and finely chopped
250g fresh wholemeal breadcrumbs
250g Roquefort cheese, crumbled
75g cashew nuts, ground

1 Preheat the oven to 190°C/gas 5.

2 Brush the mushrooms all over with olive oil and place on a baking tray.

3 Heat 3 tablespoons olive oil in a pan and gently fry the onion until soft.

4 Transfer the onions to a bowl and add the breadcrumbs, Roquefort and cashew nuts. Bind with the rest of the olive oil and use the mixture to fill the prepared mushrooms.

5 Bake for 15 minutes until cooked through and crisp on top, then serve at once.

Suggestions

Add some chopped fresh herbs to the stuffing mix.
Use houmous in place of the ground cashew nuts, using less olive oil to bind.

LENTIL FALAFEL WITH TAHINI SAUCE

Lentils do not usually need to be soaked overnight but it is essential for this recipe, Once that is done, however, the falafel only take about 10 minutes to prepare and cook. Serve this dish as a first course on a bed of rocket or as part of a mixed meze.

Makes 12

125g red or green split lentils
250ml water
½ small red onion, peeled and finely chopped
1cm fresh root ginger, peeled and grated
1 handful fresh coriander to taste
2–3 tbsp water
extra virgin olive oil, for frying
For the tahini sauce
3 tbsp tahini paste
juice of ½ lemon
1–2 tbsp water

1 Soak the lentils in the water overnight.

2 Start by making the tahini sauce. Place the tahini paste in a mug or small basin and stir in the lemon juice and a little of the water. The mixture will first thicken and then start to soften into a thick cream. Keep adding water very slowly until you reach a thick but runny cream. Keep on one side until required.

3 When you are ready to cook the falafel, drain the lentils very well and transfer to a food processor. Add the onion, ginger and fresh coriander and 2 tablespoons water.

4 Process until the mixture turns to a thick paste, stopping to scrape the

sides of the container down once or twice. You may have to rest the machine two or three times during this process. The mixture should have the texture of a soft pâté. If it is very stiff, add a little more water.

5 Heat the olive oil in a thermostatically controlled deep-fat fryer or a deep heavy-based pan to 180°C.

6 Shape the falafel paste into small flattish rounds using two table-spoons. Lower six into the hot oil and cook for 2 minutes until well browned.

7 Remove and drain on kitchen paper while you cook the remaining falafel. Serve hot or cold with the tahini.

GOAT'S CHEESE AND CHUTNEY FILO PARCELS

These little parcels make a good starter to a special meal. Serve with rocket and pea shoot salad tossed in extra virgin olive oil vinaigrette with a touch of mustard.

Serves 4

4 sheets filo pastry, about 34 × 24cm
2 tbsp extra virgin olive oil
2 small soft goat's cheese with no rind
4 heaped tsp Mango Chutney (see page 157)

1 Preheat the oven to 180°C/gas 4.

2 Place a sheet of filo pastry on a board, brush all over with olive oil and fold over once. Brush with more oil and fold again so that you have a four-layer square of pastry.

3 Place a quarter of the goat's cheese in the centre of the square and top with a heaped teaspoon of mango chutney. Gather up the corners of

the square of filo pastry and press together to form a small round parcel. Brush well all over with more olive oil and pinch the pastry together at the top of the parcel.

4 Repeat this process with three more sheets of filo pastry to make four parcels. Place in the oven and bake for 10 minutes until the parcels are lightly browned and crispy.

Suggestions for different fillings

Smoked salmon chopped with cream cheese and paprika pepper.
White crab meat mixed with ricotta cheese, grated ginger and spring onion.
Roquefort creamed with mashed potato and chopped watercress.

MAIN COURSE DISHES

PENNE WITH BROCCOLI PESTO

This is a really interesting variation on the pesto theme. It is particularly suitable for tubular pasta such as penne or rigatoni but also goes well with fusilli or orecchiette. For the most healthy dishes, choose wholegrain pasta. Save the stalks from the broccoli and use up in soups or mixed vegetable bakes or casseroles.

Serves 4

350g tubular pasta, such as penne
400g broccoli or calabrese
2 large sprigs fresh basil
2 large sprigs fresh parsley
1 small garlic clove, peeled and chopped
75g pine nuts
about 150ml extra virgin olive oil
75g Parmesan cheese, freshly grated
salt and freshly ground black pepper

1 Cook the pasta in plenty of boiling salted water, as directed on the packet, until just cooked or *al dente*.

2 Cut the florets from the broccoli and place in a blender or food processor with the basil, parsley, garlic and pine nuts. With the motor running, gradually drizzle in the olive oil until the mixture is smooth and the thick.

3 Drain the pasta and turn into a serving bowl.

4 Stir the Parmesan into the pesto, then spoon it over the pasta. Serve at once.

Healthy Highlights

The undisputed co-star in this dish is the broccoli, which is rich in glucosinolates. Broccoli has been described as a 'superfood' thanks to the antioxidant and anti-inflammatory properties of these sulphur compounds shown in many studies. In a similar way to the polyphenols in extra virgin olive oil, these effects may protect us from cancers and heart disease.

PASTA WITH TOASTED SEEDS AND FETA CHEESE

This is a lovely pasta dish with a difference. The seeds give an attractive crunchy texture and the feta provides a creamy tang.

Serves 4

400g pasta, such as penne or shells
2 tbsp pumpkin seeds
2 tbsp pine nuts
2 tbsp sesame seeds
6 tbsp extra virgin olive oil

grated zest of 1 lemon

juice of 2 lemons

20 Kalamata olives, pitted and halved

250g feta cheese, crumbled

salt and freshly ground black pepper

1 Cook the pasta in plenty of boiling salted water, as directed on the packet, until just cooked or *al dente*.

2 Toss the pumpkin seeds, pine nuts and sesame seeds in a dry frying pan over a medium heat until they are well browned and popping. Set on one side.

3 Drain the pasta and return it to the pan. Drizzle with the olive oil and toss to coat. Return to the heat and add the lemon zest, juice, olives and feta cheese. Season with pepper.

4 Serve at once topped with the seed mixture.

CAVATELLI WITH BROAD BEANS AND PEAS

This pasta recipe is very quick and easy to make, but tastes really wonderful. Look out for new season broad beans and use them as they are without skinning. Later in the year, or if you are using frozen beans, then they are better skinned.

Serves 4

300g shelled fresh broad beans

4 tbsp extra virgin olive oil

1 small onion, peeled and chopped

1 garlic clove

1 fresh red chilli, finely chopped

100g peas
2–3 tbsp vegetable stock or water
400 g cavatelli pasta
200g ricotta cheese, crumbled
30g fresh mint, roughly chopped
salt

1 Blanch the broad beans in lightly salted boiling water. Drain the beans, then refresh in ice-cold water, then dry and peel them, if needed.

2 Heat the oil in a saucepan and gently fry the onion, garlic and chilli until soft. Add the broad beans and peas with the vegetable stock or water and cook gently until the liquid has evaporated and the vegetables are tender, about 5 minutes.

3 Meanwhile, cook the pasta in plenty of boiling salted water, as directed on the packet, until just cooked or *al dente*. Drain and mix directly in the pan with the broad bean sauce.

4 Just before serving, sprinkle with the fresh ricotta cheese and mint leaves. Serve with extra virgin olive oil on the side, as usual.

GREEK CHEESE FRITTERS WITH A BEETROOT MEDLEY

Serve these two complementary dishes with bulgur mixed with chopped pistachio nuts.

Serves 2

100g Greek halloumi cheese, finely diced
75g Greek feta cheese, crumbled
4 tbsp plain flour
2 tbsp milk

3–4 tbsp chopped fresh coriander
¼ tsp ground cumin or cumin seeds, toasted in a dry pan
1 egg, beaten
extra virgin olive oil, for frying
For the beetroot medley
1 tbsp extra virgin olive oil
300g red beetroot tops
150g beetroot (2 small)
grated zest and juice of 1 small orange
freshly ground black pepper

1 Start with the beetroot medley. Heat the olive oil in a saucepan and add the beet tops. Leave to wilt over a low heat.

2 Add the diced beetroot, orange zest and rind and season with pepper. Bring to the boil and stir to heat through while you make the fritters.

3 To make the fritters, mix together the cheeses, flour, milk, herbs, pepper and egg.

4 Heat the oil in a frying pan and fry dollops of the mixture for about 3–4 minutes until lightly browned on one side. Turn and fry on the second side until lightly browned.

5 Serve at once with the beetroot.

Healthy Highlights

Beetroot is a unique source of phytonutrients called betalains. One of these, betanin has been the subject of studies which have shown significant antioxidant and anti-inflammatory effects. As with many fat-soluble vitamins and antioxidants, the absorption of similar compounds has been shown to be much enhanced as they combine with the olive oil.

GREEK GIGANTAS BEANS WITH CORIANDER

These lovely Greek beans are similar to butter beans and the latter can be used in this recipe if you can't find them. Using canned beans considerably shortens the time it takes to make the recipe, but the texture is not the same. Do not add salt to the cooking water as this tends to harden the beans. Serve this hearty dish with feta crumbled onto slices of wholemeal bread and toasted under the grill.

Serves 4

100g dried gigantas beans
6 tbsp extra virgin olive oil
200g small tomatoes
2 small onions, peeled and finely chopped
2 tbsp chopped fresh coriander
2–3 tbsp white wine
freshly ground black pepper

1 Place the beans in a saucepan and cover with plenty of water. Bring to the boil. Remove any scum which forms. Cover with a lid and reduce the heat so that the beans are just simmering. Continue cooking for about 1½–2 hours, topping up with boiling water if necessary. When the beans are cooked, drain and keep on one side.

2 Preheat the oven to 200°C/gas 6 and line a baking tray with foil. Drizzle 2 tablespoons of the olive oil onto the tray.

3 Cut the tomatoes in half horizontally and place on the tray. Bake in the oven for about 20 minutes until they begin to brown a little. Remove from the heat and scrape the centres of the tomatoes out into a bowl, discarding the skins.

4 Heat the remaining olive oil and fry the onions for about 2–3 minutes until they begin to soften. Add the skinned tomatoes and continue cooking for a further 2–3 minutes. Add half the coriander and the cooked beans. Stir and add the wine. Bring the mixture to the boil and cook for another minute.

5 Stir in the remaining coriander, season with pepper and serve at once with more extra virgin olive oil on the side to finish the dish.

LEBANESE AUBERGINE CASSEROLE

This Middle Eastern-inspired casserole is very versatile. Eat hot with bulgur or brown rice, cold as a first course or serve as part of a mixed meze meal with pitta bread.

Serves 4

4 small or 2 medium aubergines
1 onion, peeled
2 ripe tomatoes, peeled
4 garlic cloves, peeled
100g cooked or canned chickpeas, drained
3 sundried tomatoes, chopped
4 tbsp chopped fresh parsley
100ml tomato juice
4 tbsp extra virgin olive oil
¼ teaspoon ground cinnamon
freshly ground black pepper

1 Cut the aubergines lengthways so that they are not quite cut through. Arrange in a deep pan with a lid. The aubergines should be fairly tightly packed.

2 Cut the onion and tomato into four rounds horizontally. Place a slice of onion, a slice of tomato and a clove of garlic in the slit in each small aubergine or along the slit in the large ones.

3 Sprinkle with the chickpeas, sundried tomatoes and parsley. Pour on the tomato juice and olive oil. Sprinkle with cinnamon and pepper.

4 Bring to the boil. Reduce the heat, cover with a lid and simmer for 40 minutes. Remove the lid from the pan and continue to cook gently for further 15 minutes to reduce the juices.

Suggestion

Use a little less tomato juice and top with sliced potatoes. Bake in the oven at 180°C/gas 4 for about an hour to make an Aubergine Hotpot.

Healthy Highlights

Here, cinnamon gives added spice, and the cinnamaldehyde, which gives it its unique smell and taste, may have beneficial effects on blood clotting and have antimicrobial activity. Cooked with a lid, using the principles of a tagine cooking pot, means that nutrients will be retained in the dish. Sesame contains many minerals and specific lignan antioxidants such as sesamin and phytosterols which have been shown to lower cholesterol.

SPINACH-WRAPPED NUT ROAST WITH
CHILLI YOGURT SALSA

Any kind of large green leaves such as spinach, cabbage or Swiss chard can be used in this recipe. If you choose Swiss chard, cut out the stalks and use them in place of the celery. This nut roast is also delicious served cold with a salad.

Serves 6

6 large green leaves, such as spinach
30ml extra virgin olive oil
1 large onion, peeled and finely chopped
1 large garlic clove, peeled and finely chopped
1 stick celery, finely chopped
1 small aubergine, finely diced
100g carrots, peeled and grated
150g mixed ground nuts, such as Brazil nuts, walnuts and hazelnuts
100g wholemeal breadcrumbs
2 tbsp finely chopped fresh parsley
1 tbsp finely chopped fresh basil
1 tsp dried oregano
1 large egg, beaten
juice of 1 lemon
freshly ground black pepper
For the chilli salsa
4 tbsp finely chopped red onions
4 tbsp finely chopped cucumber
2 small fresh red chillis, seeded and finely chopped
juice of 2 lemons
125ml Greek yogurt

1 Preheat the oven to 180°C/gas 4. Grease and line a 900g loaf tin with olive oil and baking paper.

2 Blanch the green leaves by covering with boiling water, then plunging into cold water. Cut out the stalks and dry on kitchen paper. Use the leaves to line the prepared loaf tin.

3 Heat the olive oil for the nut loaf in a large frying pan and fry the onions, garlic and celery for 3–4 minutes until slightly softened. Add the aubergine and continue cooking over a medium heat, stirring from time to time until soft. Stir in the grated carrots and keep on one side.

4 If necessary, grind the nut mixture in a food processor, then place in a large bowl with the breadcrumbs. Stir in the vegetable mixture and all the other ingredients.

5 Spoon into the spinach-lined loaf tin. Bake for about an hour until a skewer inserted in the centre comes out clean.

6 Finally make the chilli salsa by mixing all the ingredients in a bowl.

7 To serve, turn out the nut roast onto a large serving plate and cut into thick slices. Hand round the salsa separately with some extra virgin olive oil.

SPICY SEAFOOD STIR-FRY WITH NOODLES

This is very quick to cook and mades a great dish when you are in a hurry. You can use any kind of dry noodles, but wholewheat and buckwheat noodles are the best choices.

Serves 4

125g dry noodles
2 tbsp extra virgin olive oil

2 carrots, peeled and thinly sliced on the slant

1 tbsp grated fresh root ginger

300g monkfish, cut off the bone and into small chunks

½–1 tsp Szechuan or chilli pepper

½ tsp five-spice powder

75g thin French beans

175g large peeled prawns

8 spring onions, sliced

1 tbsp white wine

splash of soy sauce

a few sprigs fresh flatleaf parsley, to garnish

1 Start by preparing the noodles as directed on the pack. Once cooked, toss in a little extra virgin olive oil and keep them warm.

2 Next, heat the remaining olive oil in a wok or deep-sided frying pan and stir-fry the carrots and ginger for 2 minutes. Add the monkfish, Szechuan or chilli pepper and five-spice powder and stir-fry for a further 3–4 minutes.

3 Add all the remaining ingredients, including the cooked noodles, and toss together for 1–2 minutes so that everything is heated through. Serve at once, garnished with parsley.

Suggestion

Use scallops in place of monkfish.

Healthy Highlights

Many Asian dishes combine spices such as chilli and ginger. Especially when cooked with olive oil, the final fusion of ingredients can be a powerful antioxidant combination. The heat in chilli derives from capsaicin which has anti-inflammatory and even pain-relieving effects, so is of particular interest in relation to arthritis. Meanwhile ginger contains gingerol which also has anti-inflammatory properties as well as regulating the digestive system.

TUNA WITH GARLIC AND CHILLI BEANS

For the best results, ask your fishmonger to cut the tuna fillets very thinly. Cook them very quickly, placing the pieces of fish in the hot frying pan and turning over the first piece as soon as you put the last piece in the pan. There should be a thin line of raw fish running through the centre of each fillet. Vincotto is a sweet condiment popular in southern Italy. It is made by boiling unfermented grape juice until it is thick and syrupy. If you can't find vincotto, use balsamic vinegar.

Serves 2

225–350g green beans, stringed if necessary
100ml extra virgin olive oil
2–3 garlic cloves, peeled and finely chopped
1 small red chilli pepper, seeded and finely chopped
200g tuna fillet, thinly sliced
a dash of vincotto or balsamic vinegar of Modena
a few fresh basil leaves

1 Steam the beans until *al dente* or almost tender.
2 Heat half the olive oil and fry the garlic until lightly browned but do not allow it to burn. Add the chopped chilli and quickly fry for

1 minute. Add the beans and toss all together for another 1–2 minutes.

3 Brush both sides of each tuna fillet slice with olive oil.

4 Heat a heavy-based pan until really hot. Cook the tuna fillet slices very quickly for about 30 seconds on each side, allowing the centre to remain raw.

5 Place the beans on warmed plates and top with the tuna slices. Add a dash of vincotto or balsamic vinegar and drizzle with the remaining oil. Garnish with fresh basil leaves.

COD IN A PARCEL WITH NOODLES

Flat noodles are often cooked in this way in northern Italy and they make a good base for all kinds of white fish fillets or steaks. Vegetarians can use sliced Fontina cheese instead of cod. It makes a good all-in-one dish to make in a hurry.

Serves 4

225g dried fettuccine or thin flat noodles
6 tbsp extra virgin olive oil
2 garlic cloves, peeled and crushed
1 small fresh chilli, seeded and finely chopped
500g ripe tomatoes, peeled and diced
1 tbsp tomato purée
12–14 pitted black olives
1 tbsp capers (optional)
200g can anchovy fillets, drained
4 cod or haddock steaks or fillets, each cut into 2–3 pieces
2 tbsp chopped fresh corianderfreshly ground black pepper

1 Preheat the oven to 200°C/gas 6 and line individual tart tins with foil, leaving plenty to fold over the top.

2 Partially cook the noodles in plenty of lightly salted boiling water for about 3–5 minutes.

3 Meanwhile, heat the oil in a saucepan and fry the garlic and chilli for 2–3 minutes. Add the tomatoes, tomato purée, olives and capers and cook for 10 minutes over a medium heat, stirring all the time.

4 Drain the pasta well and divide among the prepared tins. Top with the sauce, the anchovies and then the pieces of fish. Close up the foil parcels, leaving a fairly large space above the ingredients so that the steam can circulate inside.

5 Bake for about 15 minutes until both the pasta and the fish are just cooked.

6 Open up the parcels at the table, sprinkle with the pepper and chopped coriander and eat from the foil.

FISH CAKES WITH BEETROOT AND DILL SALSA

This is a good way to use some of the cheaper fish on sale, such as pollock, but the recipe is very good with cod or salmon too. You can buy vacuum packs of cooked beetroot which save time on preparation.

Serves 4

450g potatoes
1–2 tbsp extra virgin olive oil
450g white fish fillets, skinned if necessary
4 tbsp milk
4 tbsp water
4–6 spring onions, finely chopped

2 tbsp sesame seeds

4 tbsp fine breadcrumbs

extra virgin olive oil, for frying

For the beetroot and dill salsa

350g beetroot, cooked and finely diced

½ small red onion, peeled and finely chopped

1 small bunch fresh dill, chopped

2 tbsp extra virgin olive oil

2 tsp lemon juice

1 Cook the potatoes in boiling water until tender. Peel and mash with a fork. Stir in the olive oil to taste and keep on one side.

2 Cook the fish fillets in a little milk and water in a frying pan for about 3–5 minutes, depending on the thickness of the fillet, turning over once. Drain the fish well and check there are no bones. Flake the fish and mix with the mashed potato and spring onions. Leave the mixture to cool.

3 Make the salsa by mixing the beetroot with all the other ingredients in a bowl. Leave to stand until required.

4 Shape the fish and potato mixture into into large cakes. Mix the sesame seeds and breadcrumbs in a shallow bowl and coat the fishcakes in the mixture.

5 Heat a little oil and fry the fishcakes for about 8–10 minutes until light golden on both sides. Serve with the beetroot salsa.

SEA BASS WITH BANANAS AND TARRAGON CARROTS

The best bananas to use for this delicious combination are the small bananas from Madeira and the Canary Islands. However, larger Caribbean and other bananas can be used instead.

Serves 4

4 good-sized sea bass or other white fish fillets, skinned
120ml extra virgin olive oil
6 small or 4 large bananas, peeled and cut in half lengthways
juice of 1 lemon
plenty of coarsely ground black pepper
For the tarragon carrots
4 tbsp water
6 tbsp extra virgin olive oil
400g carrots, peeled and thinly sliced
4 sprigs fresh tarragon, chopped
freshly ground black pepper

1 Start by preparing the carrots. Pour the water and oil into a saucepan and bring to the boil. Add the carrots, tarragon and plenty of freshly ground black pepper. Cover with a lid. Cook for about 20 minutes until the carrots are very tender, then remove the lid and boil off any remaining liquid.

2 Season the fish all over with black pepper.

3 Heat the oil in a heavy-based frying pan and fry the fish on each side for about 2–3 minutes, depending on the thickness of the fillets. When you turn the fish fillets over, add the banana halves and continue frying together until the fish is cooked.

4 Transfer to serving plates and sprinkle with lemon juice. Serve with the carrots.

SALMON WITH POACHED
LEEKS AND HERBY RICE

This is a lovely combination but leeks cooked in this way are also very good served as a side dish for grilled meats and other fish or served cold with a squeeze of lemon or vinegar.

Serves 4

400g leeks
120ml extra virgin olive oil
400g salmon, skinned
freshly ground black pepper
For the herby rice
200g long-grain rice
1 onion, peeled and finely chopped
2 tsp extra virgin olive oil
400ml water
6 tbsp chopped fresh mixed herbs
freshly ground black pepper

1 Cut the leeks in half and then cut in half lengthways. Lay cut-side down in a shallow frying pan and pour on the olive oil. Place over a medium heat and as soon as the oil starts to sizzle, reduce the heat as low as possible and cover with a lid. Leave to poach for 15 minutes.

2 Meanwhile, make the herby rice. Place the rice, onion and olive oil in a saucepan and stir over a high heat for 1 minute. Add the water, stir and bring to the boil. Stir once again and cover with a lid. Reduce the heat to low and cook for 13–14 minutes until the rice is cooked and all the liquid has been absorbed. Stir in the fresh herbs and black pepper.

3 After the leeks have been poaching for 15 minutes, place the pieces of salmon on top and sprinkle with black pepper. Replace the lid and leave to cook for 10 minutes, turning the pieces of fish once.

4 To serve, spoon the rice onto serving dishes and top with the leeks and salmon and their juices.

SALMON WITH GINGER AND SPRING ONIONS ON A BED OF RAINBOW CHARD

All kinds of beet tops and chard are now available in the shops and they make a great bed on which to serve fish. If you prefer to use spinach, cut the cooking time to around 5 minutes. This recipe makes enough for a single serving, so simply multiply the ingredients by the number of people you are feeding.

Serves 1

150g salmon steak or fillet, skinned
1cm fresh root ginger, peeled and grated
½ thick continental spring onion or 3–4 small ones, thinly sliced
3 tbsp extra virgin olive oil
150g rainbow chard, Swiss chard or beet tops, washed and
    dried
To serve
lightly crushed new potatoes sprinkled with sesame seeds

1 If you have a steamer large enough to hold a plate use this, if not take the plate and place over a pan of boiling water.

2 Brush the salmon with a little of the olive oil and place on the plate. Spread the grated ginger over the fish and top with the chopped spring

onions. Pour 2 tablespoons of the olive oil over the top of the salmon. Cover with an upturned soup bowl.

3 For large quantities, use larger plate and a frying pan of boiling water. Cover with a large pan lid or shallow casserole. Leave to steam for 12–15 minutes until the fish is just cooked. The time will vary depending on the thickness of the fish.

4 Place the remaining oil in another pan and add the chard or beet tops. Cover with a lid and leave to wilt over a low heat. This will also take about 12–15 minutes. When the vegetables have reached the texture you like, remove the lid and boil off any liquid in the base of the pan.

5 Spoon the chard onto a serving plate and top with the salmon and all its juices. Serve with lightly crushed new potatoes sprinkled with sesame seeds.

CHICKEN CASSEROLE WITH TOMATOES AND GREEN OLIVES

This delicious recipe from the beautiful island of St Lucia makes an excellent all-in-one-meal. Double up if you are having a group of friends to supper.

Serves 4

2–3 garlic cloves, peeled and crushed

2 tsp red wine vinegar

1.4kg chicken, skinned and cut into 8 pieces

4 tbsp extra virgin olive oil

2 large onions, peeled and sliced

225g long-grain rice

225g can tomatoes

25g raisins

1 whole hot red chilli pepper

1 small bunch fresh chives, snipped

1 tbsp chopped fresh thyme or 1 teaspoon dried thyme

12 green olives, pitted

750ml boiling water

To serve

rice, bulgur or quinoa

1 Mix together the garlic and vinegar and rub all over the chicken pieces.

2 Heat the oil in a large saucepan and fry the chicken pieces until browned.

3 Add all the remaining ingredients and bring to the boil. Cover with a lid and simmer gently for about 35 minutes, or until the water has been absorbed and rice is tender. Stir occasionally to prevent sticking.

4 Remove the hot chilli pepper before serving with rice, bulgur or quinoa.

NORMANDY CHICKEN CASSEROLE

The prunes give a really rich character to this dish from north-west France. Olive oil was probably not the fat of choice in this region but it does give an extra dimension to the dish. There is no need to peel the apple.

Serves 4

2 heaped tbsp plain flour

1 tsp allspice

1 tsp freshly ground black pepper

8 thigh joints or 4 chicken breasts or leg joints, skinned

4 tbsp extra virgin olive oil

1 large onion, peeled and sliced

finely chopped zest of ½ lemon

300ml dry Normandy cider

150ml chicken stock

12g prunes, soaked in water overnight

1 tsp juniper berries, lightly crushed

For the garnish

2 apples, cored and sliced into rings

2 tbsp extra virgin olive oil

1 Mix together the flour, allspice and pepper, then dust the chicken portions with the seasoned flour.

2 Heat the oil in a deep frying pan with a lid. Add the chicken joints and fry for 3–4 minutes until evenly coloured on all sides. Remove from the pan and keep them warm.

3 Add the onion and lemon zest to the pan and fry for a further 2–3 minutes. Add the cider and chicken stock and bring to the boil. Return the chicken pieces to the pan. Cover with a lid and simmer for 20 minutes.

4 Next, add the prunes and juniper berries and continue to simmer for a further 20–30 minutes until the chicken is cooked through and tender.

5 Towards the end of the cooking time, slice the apple and fry in extra virgin olive oil until lightly browned on both sides. Spoon the fried apple rings and any juice onto the chicken and serve at once.

MOORISH CHICKEN WITH ORANGE AND LIME AND CORIANDER BULGUR

This dish can be cooked on the top of the stove or in the oven. The latter will take a little longer but is a useful option if you want to serve it with roasted vegetables or sweet potatoes baked in their jackets instead of bulgur.

Serves 4

8 boned chicken thighs, skinned and cut into 8 pieces
5 tbsp extra virgin olive oil
juice of 2 oranges, skins reserved and cut in half
juice of 2 limes
4 tbsp chicken or vegetable stock
4 tbsp white wine
2 tbsp capers
2 tbsp raisins
2 tbsp pine nuts or flaked almonds, toasted in a dry pan
½ tsp ground cinnamon
freshly ground black pepper
60–65g quick-cook wholewheat bulgur
50g bunch fresh coriander
50g bunch fresh parsley

1 Preheat the oven to 200°C/gas 6 if using.

2 Fry the chicken in hot olive oil until lightly browned all over. Pour in the fruit juices and the squeezed orange skins. Add the stock, wine, capers, raisins and nuts and sprinkle with cinnamon and black pepper. Bring to the boil and cover with a lid.

3 If cooking on the top of the stove, reduce the heat and simmer for about 20–25 minutes until the chicken pieces are cooked through.

4 If cooking in the oven, bake for about 25–30 minutes and check that the chicken is cooked through to the centre.

5 Prepare and cook the bulgur as set out on page 188. Process the herbs in a food processor, taking care not to chop the herbs too finely. Stir into the hot bulgur, then spoon it onto a serving plate.

6 Arrange the pieces of chicken on the top of the bulgur and spoon over all the juices.

BAKED CHICKEN WITH PEPPERS

Any strongly flavoured herbs can be used for this recipe. Rosemary, oregano and lemon thyme are all good choices. Espelette peppers come from the Basque region of France and have a very distinctive taste. However, you could use hot paprika or cayenne pepper instead. Serve with Herb Muffins (see page 269).

Serves 4

2 garlic cloves, peeled and crushed
½ tsp dried mixed herbs or 4–5 sprigs fresh herbs
grated zest and juice of 1 lemon
4 red peppers, seeded and chopped
2 tbsp olive oil
2 tbsp white wine
1 chicken, cut into about 8 portions
1 tsp clear honey
1 tsp espelette pepper
freshly ground black pepper

1 Mix the crushed garlic, the chosen herbs, the lemon zest, peppers, oil

and wine and season with pepper. Toss the chicken pieces in this mixture and leave to stand until required.

2 Preheat the oven to 200°C/gas 6 and line a baking tin with foil.

3 Arrange the chicken pieces on the foil and sprinkle with the marinade. Bake for 30 minutes until the chicken is cooked through.

4 Just before serving, mix the honey and lemon juice and drizzle over the cooked chicken. Finally sprinkle with the espelette pepper.

DUCK WITH ASPARAGUS AND FRIED NOODLES

The oriental flavours work well in this duck dish. Take care not to over-cook the duck as it may go tough.

Serves 4

250g Chinese or Japanese dry noodles

6 tbsp extra virgin olive oil

12 spring onions, sliced lengthways

2 large garlic cloves, peeled and crushed

4cm fresh root ginger, peeled and grated

200g asparagus tips

200g green beans, topped and tailed

4 tbsp water

100g piece sweet red pepper, seeded and cut into strips

4 slices duck breast or 2 large duck breasts, skinned and cut into strips

300g beansprouts

4 tsp soy sauce

1 Place the noodles in a pan and cover with boiling water. Leave to stand for 5 minutes, then place on the hob and bring to the boil or

follow the instructions on the pack. When the noodles have softened, drain well.

2 Heat 2 tablespoons olive oil in a small frying pan and add the noodles, patting them down into a flat cake. Cook over a high heat until the noodles are brown and crisp on the base. Turn over and brown the other side.

3 Heat the remaining olive oil in a wok or deep frying pan. When the oil is hot but not smoking, add the spring onions, garlic and ginger and fry for 1 minute.

4 Add the asparagus and beans and stir-fry for about 3 minutes, adding the water after a minute or so.

5 Next add the strips of red pepper and duck and continue stir-frying for 2–3 minutes until the duck is pink in the centre. Quickly add the beansprouts and soy sauce. Toss well and serve at once on a bed of the crisply fried noodles.

DUCK WITH APPLE AND LIME QUINOA

The longer you can leave the duck in the marinade the better, but even half an hour will add to the flavour. After marinating the duck, this is a very quick dish to prepare. Both the quinoa and the duck can be cooked in about 20–25 minutes. Serve with a green vegetable such as broccoli or spinach.

Serves 2

1 lime
6 tbsp extra virgin olive oil
1 star anise, slightly crushed (optional)
2 slices duck breast or 1 large duck breast, skinned

6 spring onions, thinly sliced

1 tbsp raisins

60g quinoa

150ml vegetable stock

1 apple, cored and diced

your choice of vegetables, to serve

1 Cut the lime in half and squeeze out the juice, retaining the skins. Pour the juice into a bowl with 4 tablespoons olive oil and the star anise, if using. Place the duck in this marinade and leave until it is time to cook the meal, turning from time to time.

2 To cook the quinoa, fry the spring onions in 1 tablespoon of the remaining olive oil until very lightly browned. Add the raisins and quinoa and continue frying gently for 1 minute. Add the stock and bring the mixture to the boil. Cover with a lid, reduce the heat and cook over a low heat for 15 minutes until all the liquid has been absorbed.

3 Meanwhile, cut the zest from the lime skins and slice into thin strips. Heat the last of the oil in a frying pan and fry the zest with the apple cubes for about 3–4 minutes until the apples begin to soften. Do not allow the apple to cook fully or it will go mushy. Remove the mixture from the pan and put to one side.

4 Next, heat the pan from frying the apples and when it is very hot add the duck slices or breast together with just a little of the marinade. Cook very quickly on both sides to lightly brown. Reduce the heat and continue frying for about 6–5 minutes, depending on the thickness of the meat, turning from time to time. Baste with the marinade towards the end of the cooking time. When the duck is cooked to your satisfaction, remove from the pan and leave to rest for 3 minutes.

5 Stir the apples into the quinoa, place the rested duck on top and pour the pan juices over. Add the vegetables of your choice on the side.

LAMB CUTLETS WITH SPICED BEETROOT

Just as in the previous recipe, half an hour in the marinade is worth it to add flavour to the meat, but if you can leave it longer, then that's even better. Capers, which are packed in brine or in salt crystals, need to have the salt removed by soaking in a couple of changes of water.

Serves 2

6 small lamb cutlets

3 tablespoons extra virgin olive oil

juice and grated zest of ½ lemon

1 garlic clove, peeled and crushed

1 heaped tablespoon capers, chopped

1 tsp dried oregano

For the spiced beetroot

6 tbsp extra virgin olive oil

1 tsp cumin seeds

1 tsp paprika

2 large tomatoes, peeled and finely chopped

1 large cooked beetroot, peeled and diced

1 Marinate the cutlets in a mix of olive oil, lemon juice and zest, garlic, capers and oregano. Leave to stand until you are ready to cook them.

2 Meanwhile, prepare the spiced beetroot. Heat 2 tablespoons olive oil in a pan and add the cumin seeds. They should pop and brown. Add the paprika, stir and then add the tomatoes. Stir again and add the beetroot. Cover and cook over a low heat for about 1 hour or more until the tomatoes have formed a thick sauce.

3 Remove the cutlets from the marinade. Heat a non-stick frying pan until very hot, put the cutlets in the pan and quickly brown both sides

of the meat. Add half the marinade to the pan and continue cooking the cutlets for 2–3 minutes. Add the rest of the marinade to the cutlets and boil down quickly.

4 Serve the cutlets with the remaining juices poured over the top and the spiced beetroot on the side.

Healthy Highlights

Beetroot, with its antioxidant phytonutrients, is a powerhouse for health, and in this recipe the spices add further benefits. As with many seeds, cumin is rich in minerals but it has also been studied for possible anti-cancer effects. Meanwhile paprika, along with other spices, can improve insulin sensitivity. Remember to buy small quantities of good-quality, well-reared meat to get a healthier balance of fats.

TERIYAKI BEEF WITH CITRUS NOODLES

This is a very quick dish to cook but for the best effect the meat needs to be marinated for at least 45 minutes or longer if you have the time.

Serves 2

2 minute steaks
50ml saki or dry sherry
50ml extra virgin olive oil
25ml soy sauce
1 small red onion, peeled and finely chopped
2cm fresh root ginger, peeled and grated
freshly ground black pepper

For the citrus noodles

2 tbsp sesame seeds

125g Chinese noodles

1 tbsp extra virgin olive oil

grated rind and juice of ½ orange

grated rind and juice of ½ grapefruit

100g beansprouts

1 Flatten the meat by beating with a rolling pin between two pieces of cling film. Place in a shallow dish. Mix all the remaining main ingredients and pour over the meat. Leave to stand until required.

2 To make the noodles, toast the sesame seeds in a dry frying pan or under the grill. They brown very quickly so stir regularly and keep an eye on them.

3 Plunge the noodles into a large pan of boiling water and cook or leave to stand for the length of time given on the pack. Drain and toss with all the remaining noodle ingredients over a medium heat.

4 To cook the beef, drain off the marinade and grill over a barbecue or under a hot grill for 3–4 minutes for rare steaks and for longer for medium and well-done steaks. Serve on a bed of noodles.

SPANISH MARINATED PORK WITH BEANS

This recipe comes from Extremadura in western Spain and uses the smoked pimentón of the region called Pimentón de la Vera. If you cannot find it, use hot Hungarian paprika instead. Store the marinating pork in the fridge but do not try to cut down on the time as 48 hours is essential to get the full flavour. Serve with good bread to mop up the juices and a dressed rocket and watercress salad on the side.

Serves 6

2 tbsp hot Pimentón de la Vera

175ml extra virgin olive oil

2 tsp dried oregano

2 garlic cloves, peeled and crushed

2 large pork fillets

100g dry white beans

75ml sherry

1 large onion, peeled and sliced

freshly ground black pepper

1 Preheat the oven to 180°C/gas 4.

2 Dissolve the pimentón in 75ml olive oil and add the oregano and garlic. Place the pork fillets in a shallow dish and rub all over with the pimentón mixture. Add water just to cover and place in the fridge. Leave to marinate for 48 hours.

3 Meanwhile, soak the beans in cold water overnight.

4 Preheat the oven to 180°C/gas 4.

5 Remove the meat from the marinade just before cooking and dry on kitchen paper. Heat the most of the remaining olive oil and fry the meat until lightly browned. Transfer to an ovenproof dish with a lid and pour on the sherry and about half the juices from the marinade. Bake in the oven for about 1 hour, or until the meats shows no pink colour when cut.

6 Meanwhile, drain the white beans and cook in a small amount of water for 20–30 minutes until just tender.

7 Heat the remaining olive oil in a pan and gently fry the onion until soft but not brown. Toss with the cooked beans and heat through. Season with pepper to taste.

8 Slice the meat and serve on a bed of beans and onions. Pour the pan
   juices from the meat over the top.

Healthy Highlights

Here is a great example of a marinade that not only tastes great but
also serves to protect the meat from potentially harmful effects of
changes in chemistry during the cooking process. The high antioxidant ingredients – based on the extra virgin olive oil, spices and garlic
– will coat the meat and keep potentially unhealthy HAs (see page
105) (amines) from building up during the cooking process.

DESSERTS, CAKES AND BISCUITS

FRIED BANANAS WITH MIXED SEEDS

Frying bananas in olive oil is a good way of using up bananas which have got very ripe.

Serves 2

1 tbsp pumpkin seeds
1 tbsp sunflower seeds
1 tbsp pine nuts
2 tbsp extra virgin olive oil
1cm fresh ginger root, peeled and grated
juice and zest of ½ lime
2 tbsp clear honey
4 tbsp dark rum
2 bananas, peeled and cut in half lengthways

1 Toast the seeds and pine nuts in a dry frying pan until lightly browned.
2 Heat the olive oil in pan and gently fry the ginger and lime zest for a minute or so.

3 Stir in the lime juice, honey and rum. Carefully place the banana halves in the mixture and bring to the boil. Cook over a fairly high heat for a few minutes to reduce the sauce.

4 Transfer the bananas to warmed serving plates. Sprinkle with the prepared seeds and nuts and pour the pan juices over the top. Serve at once.

Suggestion

Use lightly toasted desiccated coconut in place of the seeds.

FRENCH TOAST WITH LEMON APPLE PURÉE

It's a good idea to double up on the apples and save half the purée to use to sweeten other dishes such as Date and Walnut Muffins (see page 271).

Serves 4

For the lemon apple purée
4 large eating apples, peeled and cored
3 tbsp water
2 tbsp raisins
1 tbsp lemon juice
grated zest of ½ lemon
For the French toast
2 eggs
2 tbsp milk
¼–½ tsp five-spice powder
4 slices day-old bread
2 tbsp extra virgin olive oil

1 Place the apples in a pan with the water and bring to the boil. Reduce the heat and simmer for 15–20 minutes, stirring from time to time to ensure that the apples do not burn.

2 Meanwhile, soak the raisins in the lemon juice. When the apples are soft, mash with a fork, then stir in the raisins and lemon zest.

3 To make the French toast, beat the eggs and stir in the milk and five-spice. Place in a bowl and soak the pieces of bread in the mixture.

4 Heat the olive oil in a frying pan and fry the pieces of soaked bread on both sides until well browned and slightly crispy.

5 Arrange on a warm plate with the apple lemon purée and serve at once.

BANANA PANCAKES

These very quickly made pancakes are a kind of cross between drop scones and a sweet tortilla. Keep them small or you will not be able to turn them over. Serve with a fruit purée.

Makes 8 small pancakes

1 large banana, well mashed
1 egg
¼ tsp ground cinnamon
a very little extra virgin olive oil

1 Mix the mashed banana with the egg and cinnamon.

2 Brush a large non-stick frying pan with a little olive oil and place over a medium heat.

3 Drop small spoonfuls of the banana and egg mixture onto the hot pan. Leave to set and cook for about 2 minutes.

4 When the bases are set and well browned, turn the pancakes over and cook on the other side until well browned.

5 Serve at once on warm plates.

BRAISED PEARS WITH GINGER AND RAISINS

This useful recipe can be cooked in two different ways depending on what else you are cooking for the rest of the meal. If you are using the oven you can braise the pears at the same time. If you are cooking on the top of the stove the pears can be cooked in a shallow pan with a lid. The cooking times and temperatures will need to be adjusted accordingly.

Serves 4

4 hard pears, peeled, cored and quartered
75g raisins
3 tbsp extra virgin olive oil
2 tbsp sherry
juice of 1 lemon
grated zest of ½ lemon
1cm fresh root ginger, finely grated

1 Preheat the oven to 170°C/gas 3.

2 Place the pears and raisins in an ovenproof dish with a lid or in the chosen saucepan. Add all the remaining ingredients.

3 If baking, cover with a lid and bake for about 1 hour until the pears are tender.

4 If cooking on the top of the stove, cover with a lid and carefully bring the liquid to the boil. Reduce the heat almost to the lowest setting

DESSERTS, CAKES AND BISCUITS

and simmer very gently for about 1 hour in a shallow pan and about 2 hours in a deeper pan, turning the pears in the latter from time to time.

PLUMS WITH ALMOND CRUMBLE TOPPING

This crumble is not as crunchy as the crumble topping for the apricots on page 256 but it is equally delicious and suits the plums very well. You can add a little freshly grated ginger or a star anise to the plums for a change.

Serves 4

12 plums
100ml red wine
1 tsp grated fresh root ginger (optional)
1 star anise (optional)
For the crumble
50g wholemeal flour
50g rolled oats
15g ground almonds
50ml extra virgin olive oil
2 tbsp clear honey

1 Preheat the oven to 190°C/gas 5.

2 Cook the plums in the red wine with ginger or star anise, if using. Bring to the boil, then reduce the heat and cook for 5–15 minutes depending of the variety and ripeness of the plums.

3 Transfer to an ovenproof dish. The plum juice should come about halfway up the plums. If there is too much, keep on one side and use in fresh fruit smoothies.

4 To make the crumble, place the dry ingredients in a basin and pour on the oil and honey. Mix together with a fork. Place the crumble on top of the plums in small dollops, using a teaspoon.

5 Bake for 30 minutes until the top is lightly browned and crisp.

APRICOTS WITH SESAME CRUMBLE

The crumble topping for this dessert can be made in advance and frozen for future use with apricots or other fruits.

Serves 4

10–12 apricots, stoned
4 tbsp white wine
For the crumble
50g rolled oats
35g wholemeal flour
25g ground almonds
25g sesame seeds
2 tbsp extra virgin olive oil, plus extra for greasing
1 tbsp clear honey

1 Preheat the oven to 190°C/gas 5 and lightly grease a baking tray.

2 To make the crumble topping, place the dry ingredients in a bowl and add the oil and honey. Use your fingers to mix all the ingredients together to make a crumbly mixture. Spread out over the prepared baking tray and bake for 5 minutes. Remove from the tray and use at once or allow to cool and keep for future use.

3 Cook the apricots and the wine in a saucepan over a low heat for 8–10 minutes until tender. Transfer to an ovenproof dish and top with the semi-cooked crumble.

4 Bake for about 10 minutes until the top is lightly browned and crispy.

MAIDS OF HONOUR

These tarts take a little time to make but they are worth the effort for a special occasion. Serve with a really creamy Greek yogurt.

Makes 10 tarts

250g Shortcrust Pastry made with olive oil (see page 258)
a little flour, for dusting
For the filling
14 dried apricots, soaked overnight and cooked till tender in 3–4
    tbsp water
2 small eggs, at room temperature
1 tbsp clear honey
2 tbsp extra virgin olive oil
75g ground almonds

1 Make the pastry first as it needs to stand in the fridge for an hour before rolling out.

2 Preheat the oven to 190°C/gas 5 and line 10 individual tart tins with baking paper.

3 Mash the apricots into a thick purée.

4 Next roll out the pastry quite thinly on a lightly floured surface. Cut into 10 rounds to fit your tart tins, leaving a slight overlap, as the pastry tends to shrink a little while waiting for the filling to go in.

5 Place the eggs and honey in a bowl and beat with an electric whisk

until the mixture thickens. Gradually add the olive oil, still whisking, then fold in the ground almonds.

6 Place a small spoonful of apricot purée in the base of each tart and top with the almond mixture, working as quickly as you can.

7 Place the tarts in the oven and bake for 20–25 minutes until the filling is just set.

SHORTCRUST PASTRY

Using olive oil in place of butter produces a healthy pastry that is really crisp, though perhaps a little harder to work with. You can make a large batch, divide it up and store it in the freezer.

Makes about 475–500g pastry

225g self-raising flour (or plain flour with 3½ teaspoons baking powder)
75g plain flour
100ml extra virgin olive oil
100ml water

1 Place the flours in a large bowl and pour on the olive oil and water. Stir together with a tablespoon and finally bring together with your hands to form a large soft ball.

2 Cut the ball in half, and wrap each portion in cling film. Store in the fridge for 1 hour before using.

PROFITEROLES WITH STRAWBERRY
CREAM FILLING

Olive oil makes excellent profiteroles, which are indistinguishable from those make with butter.

Makes 12–14 profiteroles

For the profiteroles
150ml water
3 tbsp extra virgin olive oil
75g plain flour
2 eggs

For the strawberry cream filling
200g strawberries
4 heaped tbsp Greek yogurt

1 Preheat the oven to 200°C/gas 6.

2 Place the water and olive oil in a deep pan and bring to the boil. Add all the flour and beat very well with a wooden spoon. The liquid will take up the flour and form a smooth ball of dough which comes away from the sides of the pan. Leave to cool a little for 3–4 minutes.

3 Break 1 egg into the pan and beat hard with a wooden spoon until the egg is thoroughly amalgamated into the dough. Repeat the process with the second egg.

4 Pipe small blobs of the dough onto a non-stick baking tray or make small heaps with a spoon – roughly the size of a walnut.

5 Bake for 13–14 minutes until the profiteroles are a delicate golden brown. Reduce the heat to 180°C/gas 4 and continue to cook for a further 5–8 minutes to dry out the pastry.

6 Transfer to a wire rack and make a horizontal slit in each profiterole with a knife. Leave to cool. Keep away from any damp atmosphere or the profiteroles will soften.

7 To make the filling, either purée the strawberries in a blender or chop very finely and mix with the yogurt. Place small spoonfuls inside each profiterole.

CARROT CAKE

For a special occasion you can frost this cake with cream cheese mixed with a little milk and a few drops of vanilla extract.

Makes 1 large loaf (12 slices)

300ml extra virgin olive oil, plus extra for greasing
300g plain flour or half and half plain flour and wholemeal flour,
    plus extra for dusting
4 large eggs
1 tbsp baking powder
1 tsp ground cinnamon
1 pinch salt
300g carrots, peeled and finely grated
150g raisins
50g pecan nuts, chopped
2 tbsp milk

1 Preheat the oven to 190°C/gas 5 and brush a 900g loaf tin with olive oil. Shake a little flour round the inside of the tin to make a fine coating, discarding any excess.

2 Beat the eggs with the oil and sugar until very well blended. Stir in the flour, baking powder, cinnamon and salt. Carefully fold in the carrots,

raisins and nuts. Finally add the milk to make a fairly thick but dropping consistency. Pour the mixture into the prepared loaf tin and place in the oven.

3 Bake for 30 minutes, then cover with a double thickness of kitchen foil. Continue cooking for about 1–1¼ hours until cooked through. A skewer pushed into the centre should come out clean.

4 Leave to cool for 10 minutes, then remove the cake from the tin. Leave to cool on a wire rack.

Healthy Highlights

A cake with extra virgin olive oil and other healthy ingredients – like other recipes in this section there is no need to cut out delicious cake or cookie treats to follow a healthy Olive Oil Diet!

ORANGE AND PRUNE TEA BREAD

This lovely loaf is sweetened with a prune purée which needs to be made prior to cooking the loaf. It is worth making a larger quantity of purée than you need for this cake, then use the rest to make a dessert with yogurt and orange juice or to make Chocolate Layer Cake (see page 265).

Makes a 900g loaf

For the prune purée
10 large pitted prunes
For the tea bread
2 eggs

4 tbsp extra virgin olive oil, plus extra for greasing

125ml milk

125g prune purée

grated zest of 1 orange

½ tsp mixed spice or allspice

150g self-raising flour

150g wholemeal flour

1 To make the prune purée, soak the prunes in cold water overnight, then drain and simmer gently in a little fresh water for 5–8 minutes until soft. Purée in a blender or food processor. Measure out 125g to use for this tea bread.

2 Preheat the oven to 180°C/gas 4. Line a 900g loaf tin with baking paper and brush with a little olive oil.

3 Break the eggs into a mixing bowl and whisk in the olive oil, milk and 125g prune purée.

4 Mix the flours together. Gradually fold the flours into the liquid mixture. Spoon into the prepared loaf tin and bake for about 55–60 minutes until lightly browned on top and a skewer inserted in the centre comes out clean. Cook for a little longer if necessary. Turn out onto a wire rack to cool.

Suggestion

Add 2 tablespoons of raisins for a sweeter cake.

CHOCOLATE CUP CAKES

When you make a purée, it's always worth making a bit extra to use in other recipes – this apricot purée can be used in Maids of Honour (see page 257), for example. Alternatively, freeze in small quantities so you always have some ready to use.

Makes 12

For the apricot purée
225g dried apricots, soaked in cold water overnight
3 tbsp white wine
For the cup cakes
100g plain flour
30g cocoa powder
½ tsp baking powder
2 eggs
4 tbsp extra virgin olive oil
75g apricot purée
2 tbsp milk

1 Drain the apricots, reserving the liquid, then purée in a blender or food processor, adding enough of the soaking water to make a thick consistency.

2 Preheat the oven to 180°C/gas 4. Arrange 12 non-stick paper cup cases on a baking tray or in the holes of a bun tin.

3 Sift the flour, cocoa powder and baking powder into a bowl.

4 Mix the eggs, olive oil and 75g of the apricot purée in another bowl. Pour the liquid mixture into the flour and mix with a wooden spoon. Add enough milk to give a good dropping consistency.

5 Spoon the mixture into the prepared cup cases and bake for 15–20 minutes until they are cooked through. Transfer to a wire rack to cool.

6 Store in an airtight tin and eat within 3–4 days or freeze to keep the cakes for longer.

CHOCOLATE ICING

This recipe makes a nice chocolate icing, but it is not shiny.

Makes enough to coat a 20cm cake

75g dark chocolate with 70% cocoa
1 tbsp extra virgin olive oil

1 Melt the chocolate in a basin over a pan of hot water. When all the chocolate has melted, stir in the olive oil and leave to cool. This will take about 15 minutes.

2 Towards the end of that time, the mixture will start to thicken. Use the icing quickly to coat buns and cakes. The mixture starts to set quite fast at this stage.

To make truffles

If you work really fast, it is possible to catch the mixture as it is stiffening up and roll it between your fingers to make truffles. Roll at once in chopped nuts.

CHOCOLATE LAYER CAKE WITH
YOGURT AND RASPBERRIES

This rich chocolate cake can also be served on its own at tea time. For a real treat, turn the cake over and coat with Chocolate Icing (see opposite). Cut into squares to serve.

Serves 8

125g self-raising flour
50g cocoa powder
75g ground almonds
125ml extra virgin olive oil
135g prune purée (see page 261)
2 large eggs
3 tbsp strong black coffee, cooled
4 tbsp raspberries
4 tbsp thick Greek yogurt
a few squares of dark chocolate

1 Preheat the oven to 180°C/gas 4 and oil an 18cm square baking tin.

2 Sift the flour and cocoa into a large mixing bowl and stir in the ground almonds. Beat together the olive oil, prune purée, eggs and coffee and pour into the bowl together with the dry ingredients and mix well to combine.

3 Spoon the cake mixture into the prepared tin and smooth the top flat with a knife. Bake for 20 minutes until cooked through.

4 Remove from the oven, leave to cool a little, then transfer to a wire rack to cool fully. Cut the cake into 8 squares and slice horizontally through the middle.

5 Mix together the raspberries and yogurt and spread this mixture over the base pieces of cake. Top with the second halves and grate a little dark chocolate over the top.

Suggestions

Use chopped orange slices, peaches or strawberries in place of the raspberries.

Healthy Highlights

An indulgence that is part of the Olive Oil Diet! Combining the polyphenols and healthy fats of extra virgin olive oil with anti-oxidant-rich cocoa and coffee makes for an amazingly healthy alternative chocolate cake. A phytonutrient called rheosmin in raspberries appears to have a very positive effect on reducing the risk of gaining weight. Use organic raspberries when possible.

SPROUTED SODA BREAD

This recipe gives an excellent texture to the loaf. It is not as dry as some soda breads. Use short English-style beansprouts rather than the much longer Chinese beansprouts.

Makes 1 large loaf

200g plain flour, plus extra for dusting
200g wholemeal flour
50g rolled oats
50g sprouted beans or chickpeas

1 tsp baking powder

1 tsp bicarbonate of soda

275ml milk

2 tbsp extra virgin olive oil

1 tbsp lemon juice

1 Preheat the oven to 200°C/gas 6.

2 Mix all the dry ingredients in a bowl, stir well and make a well in the centre.

3 Mix the milk, olive oil and lemon juice, pour into the dry ingredients and mix together using a wooden spoon to form a dough.

4 Flour a work surface and gently knead the bread 4–5 times. Shape into a large oval and place on a floured baking tray. Flatten slightly and cut a deep cross in the centre of the loaf.

5 Bake for 30–35 minutes. Remove from the oven and cool on a wire tray. Serve warm or cold.

SAVOURY SCONES

You can vary these savoury scones by adding dried herbs or spices to the mix.

Makes 6

40ml extra virgin olive oil, plus extra for greasing

150g plain flour, plus extra for dusting

1 tbsp baking powder

100g fine oatmeal

100ml buttermilk

freshly ground black pepper

1 Preheat the oven to 200°C/gas 6 and lightly oil a baking tray.

2 Sift the flour and baking powder into a mixing bowl and stir in the oatmeal.

3 Whisk the buttermilk and oil together and pour over the dry ingredients. Mix together and knead very gently with your hands to make a soft dough.

4 Roll out the dough on a lightly floured surface to about 3–4cm thick. Cut into rounds, place on the prepared tray and bake for 10 minutes until risen and just firm.

5 Cool on a wire rack.

CHEESE MUFFINS

These light and airy muffins can be served hot or cold. They can also be served with soups and other salads instead of bread.

Makes 12

For the muffins
6 tbsp extra virgin olive oil
125g wholemeal flour
50g fine oatmeal
2 tsp baking powder
½ tsp bicarbonate of soda
1 pinch salt
100g mature Pecorino or Cheddar cheese
dried red red chilli flakes (optional)
150g thick set sheep's or goat's milk yogurt
125ml milk
1 egg, beaten

1 Preheat the oven to 200°C/gas 6 and generously oil a muffin tin.

2 Mix together the flour, oatmeal, baking powder, bicarbonate of soda and salt. In another bowl mix all the remaining ingredients.

3 Combine all the ingredients from the two bowls and spoon into the prepared muffin tins.

4 Place in the oven and bake for 20–25 minutes until light brown in colour. Remove from the oven and ease the muffins out onto a wire rack to cool.

HERB MUFFINS

These savoury muffins are great to serve in place of bread to mop up runny sauces and casseroles. Alternatively, serve warm with salads, cut in half and drizzled with extra virgin olive oil.

Makes 12

4 tbsp extra virgin olive oil, plus extra for greasing
1 onion, peeled and finely chopped
¼ tsp dried herbs or 2–3 sprigs fresh herbs
2 eggs
300ml milk
200ml plain flour
100g fine oatmeal
1½ tbsp baking powder

1 Preheat the oven to 400°C/gas 6 and generously oil a muffin tin.

2 Heat the olive oil in a pan and gently fry the onions until soft but not brown. Add the chosen herbs. Transfer to a bowl and leave to cool for a minute. Add the eggs and milk, then add all the dry ingredients and mix well together.

3 Spoon into the prepared muffin tin and bake in the oven for 20–25 minutes until risen and golden.

BLUEBERRY BREAKFAST MUFFINS

These light and fluffy muffins make a great weekend breakfast. They are very quick to make and do not need anything adding to them. They freeze well, too, so store leftover muffins – if you have any – in the freezer and warm them up quickly in a hot oven.

Makes 12

125g plain flour
125g wholemeal flour
3 tsp baking powder
200g blueberries
2 eggs
120g extra virgin olive oil
100ml milk
1 tsp vanilla extract

1 Preheat the oven to 190°C/gas 4 and generously oil a muffin tin.

2 Mix the dry ingredients and the blueberries in a bowl, crushing just a few of the blueberries with a fork.

3 Mix together all the wet ingredients, then pour over the dry ingredients. Mix, then spoon into the prepared muffin tin.

4 Bake for 25 minutes until lightly browned and cooked through to the centre.

DATE AND WALNUT MUFFINS

These muffins are particularly good served in place of scones with thick Greek yogurt and a fruit purée, such as apricot (see page 263) or apple.

Makes 12

300g wholemeal flour
150g chopped pitted dates
100g chopped walnuts
1 tbsp baking powder
1 tsp ground cinnamon
2 eggs, beaten
100g apple purée
100ml milk
75ml extra virgin olive oil

1 Preheat the oven to 375°C/gas 5 and generously oil a muffin tin.

2 Mix all the dry ingredients in a large bowl.

3 Beat the eggs with the apple purée, milk and olive oil and pour over the dry ingredients. Mix well, then spoon into the prepared muffin tin.

4 Bake for 20–25 minutes until the muffins are cooked through and a skewer inserted in the centre comes out clean.

DATE AND BANANA COOKIES

This recipe can be used to make semi-crisp cookies or a square tray bake which will be softer in texture.

Makes 12

100g rolled oats
50g wholemeal flour
100g chopped pitted dates
2 bananas
60ml extra virgin olive oil

1 Preheat the oven to 180°C/gas 4 and line a baking tray with baking paper.

2 Mix the rolled oats, flour and dates in a bowl.

3 Mash the bananas well and tip into the bowl with the olive oil. Mix all the ingredients well together and leave to stand for 15 minutes.

4 Shape the mixture into 12 balls and place, well apart, on the prepared baking tray. Push the balls flat with the back of a spoon.

5 Bake for 15–20 minutes until well cooked and browning round the edges.

6 Transfer to a wire rack to cool. The cookies will be crisp on the edges and softer in the middle.

BANANA AND WALNUT FLAPJACK

With just five minutes' preparation time, this is simplicity itself.

Makes 12 slices

3 tbsp extra virgin olive oil, plus extra for greasing
200g rolled oats
75g walnuts, roughly chopped
1 tsp ground cinnamon
1 tsp ground ginger
1 large banana
2 tbsp clear honey

1 Preheat the oven to 180°C/gas 4 and grease a 22 ×18cm flapjack tin.

2 Place all the dry ingredients in a mixing bowl.

3 Mash the banana with a fork and add to the dry ingredients with the olive oil and honey. Mix together well, then press into the base of the prepared tin. Mark into 12 portions with a knife.

4 Bake for 45 minutes until well browned round the edges. Transfer to a wire rack to cool.

GINGER BISCUITS

These simple biscuits are best eaten fairly soon after baking.

Makes 12

75ml extra virgin olive oil, plus extra for greasing
175g plain flour, plus extra for dusting
1 tsp baking powder

2 tsp freshly grated root ginger

1 tsp vanilla extract

1 tbsp clear honey

1 egg, beaten

1 Preheat the oven to 180°C/gas 4 and oil a baking sheet.

2 Sift the flour and baking powder into a bowl and stir in the grated ginger.

3 Mix the olive oil, vanilla and honey. Place the beaten egg in a measuring jug, make up to 75g with water, then add to the oil and honey and whisk well together. Add this mixture to the dry ingredients and mix with a wooden spoon. Shape into a soft ball with your hands.

4 On a floured surface, roll out the ball of dough as thinly as possible and cut into 12–15 rounds with a pastry cutter.

5 Transfer to the baking sheet and cook for about 8–9 minutes until well browned. You may need to stand over them for the last few minutes as they can burn quite quickly.

6 Leave to cool on a wire rack.

Suggestions

Use finely-chopped raisins, or ground nuts in place of the ginger.

OATCAKES

These quick and easy-to-make oatcakes are delicious in their own right but they are also great for anyone who has a problem with wheat or gluten.

Makes 16

2 tbsp extra virgin olive oil, plus extra for greasing
100g fine oatmeal
50g rolled oats
1 tsp freshly ground black pepper
1 pinch salt
75ml water
a handful of flour, for dusting

1 Preheat the oven to 170°C/gas 3 and lightly grease a baking tray.

2 Place the oatmeal in a bowl with the seasonings and mix well. Stir in the oil and the water and mix to a light dough with your hands. Add a little more oil if the mixture is too stiff. Shape into a ball.

3 Roll out on a floured surface to about 5mm thick. Using cutters or a wine glass, cut out 16 oatcakes and place on the prepared baking tray, re-rolling the trimmings as necessary.

4 Bake for 15–20 minutes until very lightly browned and crisp. Cool on a wire rack.

Healthy Highlights

Oats contain a specific kind of fibre called beta glucan which has been shown to reduce levels of the harmful type of cholesterol. Coupled with the extra virgin olive oil, these oatcakes are an excellent way to combine heart-healthy oats with olive oil.

PARMESAN AND OLIVE TWISTS

Olive oil helps to make this simple variation on cheese straws even crisper than usual. Choose good-quality olives. Avoid ready-stoned so-called 'pizza' olives as they are produced by an accelerated method using green olives which are then dyed with ferrous oxide.

Serves 4

125ml extra virgin olive oil, plus extra for greasing
50g green or black olives, pitted and finely chopped
50g Parmesan cheese, freshly finely grated
125ml white wine
275g plain flour, plus extra for dusting
freshly ground black pepper

1 Preheat the oven to 200°C/gas 6 and grease a baking tray.

2 Place the olives, cheese, olive oil and wine in a large bowl. Gradually add the flour and pepper, stirring all the time. The mixture is ready when it begins to leave the sides of the bowl and forms into a moist and pliable ball. It should not be sticky.

3 If possible, wrap in cling film and leave for an hour to rest in the fridge.

4 Place the dough on a well-floured board and roll out. This may need to be done in batches. Cut into 20–30 strips about 10cm in length and twist round to form curly sticks.

5 Place on a baking tray and bake for 20 minutes until golden brown in colour.

6 Transfer to a wire rack to cool.

CRISP ROSEMARY FLATBREAD

This flatbread is great to make even when you do not have much time. The thinner you roll the dough the crisper the flatbreads will be. I sometimes make a slightly thicker flatbread and serve drizzled with olive oil.

Makes 4

150g plain flour, plus extra for dusting
75g wholemeal flour
1 tbsp chopped fresh rosemary
1 tsp bicarbonate of soda
½ tsp salt
125ml water
75ml extra virgin olive oil

1 Preheat the oven to 220°C/gas 7 and lightly grease a baking tray.

2 Mix the two flours, chopped rosemary, bicarbonate of soda and salt in a bowl.

3 Mix the water and olive oil together. Pour this mixture into the dry ingredients and mix with a wooden spoon until a dough forms.

4 Knead it gently on a lightly floured work surface. Divide the dough into 4 small balls and cover them in cling film while you work on one at a time.

5 Roll out the balls one at a time on a lightly floured surface to make a thin round about 16cm in diameter. Place on the prepared baking tray and bake for about 6–7 minutes until golden brown, while you continue to roll out and bake the remaining balls of dough.

CRISPY POTATO CAKES

Add some hard grated cheese and snipped chives to the potato cake mixture for an even more substantial dish.

Serves 4

600g potatoes, peeled and cubed
50g fine oatmeal
2 tbsp extra virgin olive oil, plus extra for greasing
2 tbsp milk

1 Preheat the oven to 200°C/gas 6 and grease a baking tray.
2 Steam the potato cubes until tender.
3 Mash the potatoes and mix with the oatmeal, oil and milk. Transfer to the prepared baking tray and spread flat, patting down with the palm of your hand until it is about 5mm thick.
4 Bake for 15 minutes until golden brown and crispy round the edges.

POTATO DOSAS

These are great for mopping up runny dishes and sauces.

Makes 8

500g cold mashed potato
300g wholemeal flour or half and half white flour and fine oatmeal
4 tbsp extra virgin olive oil
1 tbsp dried oregano
freshly ground black pepper

1 Mix the mashed potato with the flour or flour and oatmeal with your fingers as if you were rubbing fat into flour for pastry. Work in the olive oil, herbs and pepper to make a smooth dough.

2 Divide the dough in half and roll out one batch of the dough between two layers of cling film. Roll as thinly as possible and cut into 4 squares or rounds.

3 Cook in batches in a large dry frying pan over quite a high heat. Flip the dosas over at intervals until both sides are crisp and speckled dark brown. Keep them warm while you cook the remaining dosas in the same way.

AN OLIVE OIL DIET GLOSSARY

Acidity: Acidity in olive oil refers to the free fatty acid content of the oil. Free fatty acids are formed when fat molecules start to break up.

Alphalinolenic acid: This is a polyunsaturated fatty acid also known as Omega-3. This name is sometimes shortened to linolenic acid.

Alzheimer's disease: A form of dementia characterised by a build up of protein 'plaques' and 'tangles' in the brain.

Anti-inflammatory: Something which reduces inflammation. This may describe the property of a chemical or a substance which has that effect.

Antioxidants: These are naturally occurring molecules in our food which can neutralise or 'mop up' free radicals and so repair the damage done through oxidative stress.

Arteriosclerosis: The process where fatty deposits and plaques build up on blood vessel walls resulting in diseased, hardened and thickened arteries. This increases the risk of strokes and heart attacks.

Arthritis: Arthritis is a term used to describe a range of conditions characterised by pain and inflammation in the joints.

Atoms: These form part of the make up of all molecules. Each atom has a central positively charged core called a nucleus, surrounded by circulating negatively charged pairs of electrons. The pairing of these negatively charged electrons orbiting around the positively charged nucleus makes the atom stable.

Carbohydrates: Made up of sugar and starches, these are known as simple and complex carbohydrates respectively.

Calories: This is a measurement of energy in food.

Carotene: A group of fat soluble hydrocarbon orange coloured compounds produced by plants which have been studied for their antioxidant properties.

Cholesterol: This is a compound found in most body tissues. It has a significant role in the chemistry of our cells. It is also the medium by which chemicals are carried in the blood stream from one part of the body to another. It is made up of high-density lipids and low density lipids.

Coronary heart disease: This describes the condition which is the result of diseased arteries causing a blockage or interruption to the blood supply to the heart.

Dementia: The term used to describe a group of symptoms which effect an individual's capacity to think, problem solve, recall events or express themselves.

Diabetes: This is a condition which causes a person's blood sugar level to be too high. There are different forms of diabetes. It is often associated with other illnesses and diseases.

Electrons: Atoms have a central positively charged core called a nucleus, surrounded by circulating negatively charged pairs of electrons.

Embolus: A mass of material, usually a blood clot, which causes a blockage to a blood vessel.

Exponential: An increasingly rapid rise.

Fats: These are made up of different fatty acids joined together along with some non-fatty acid components.

Fatty acids: These are complicated molecules consisting of carbon, hydrogen and oxygen atoms bound together with chemical bonds. These chemical bonds may be single or double.

Fibre: Plant substances which cannot be fully broken down by the human digestive system. They provide bulk, improve digestive health and have a beneficial effect on heart disease, body weight and in reducing the risk of some cancers.

Free radicals: These are unstable by-products of the normal ongoing chemical reactions in the body. These products consist of atoms which have lost an electron from a pair. These atoms are unstable and some will 'scavenge' electrons from other atoms in the molecules of our cellular structures.

Glyaecemic index/Glyaecemic load: The index is a unit measurement representing the effect a particular food has on blood sugar levels. The load is the measured actual effect on blood glucose of the total food or meal consumed.

Glucose: A simple sugar, or monosaccharide, which is part of the carbohydrate macronutrient group and which is a source of energy for the body.

Haemorrhage: An uncontrolled loss of blood from the circulatory system which can occur as a consequence of rupture of blood vessel wall.

Hexane: This is a chemical solvent used in the extraction of oils from seeds.

Hydrogenation: A chemical process in which hydrogen is added to the original fat molecule. It produces a hardened vegetable fat which is more easily used by the food industry.

Ibuprofen: A widely available drug used to treat inflammation and pain.

Immune system: This is the structure and processes within our bodies designed to provide defence against disease, including infectious pathogens.

Inflammatory: This is the term used to describe the state, where the immune system is involved as part of the body's response to potentially harmful stimuli. Inflammation can result from external damage or disease and internal chemical processes.

High-density lipids (HDL): This is the form of cholesterol which is considered to be beneficial.

Insulin: A hormone produced by the pancreas which regulates carbohydrates and fats. It acts to ensure safe levels of glucose are maintained and controls the storage and utilisation of energy.

Insulin sensitivity: This describes the amount of insulin required by an individual to regulate blood glucose levels. With decreasing sensitivity to the effects of insulin, a person may be said to be increasingly insulin resistant.

Legumes: A type of plant, for example beans or peas, with edible seeds that grow in cases, or pods. The pods themselves are often edible also.

Lignans: A group of plant chemicals belonging to the polyphenol class which have antioxidant properties.

Linoleic acid: This is a polyunsaturated fatty acid also known as Omega-6.

Linolenic acid: See Alphalinolenic acid.

Low-density lipids (LDL): This is the form of cholesterol which is considered to be particularly detrimental to health.

Lubricin: A particular molecule which consists of protein and carbohydrate which is present in joints and which acts as a lubricant.

Meta analyses: This is the joint analysis of several published studies to analyse the combined results.

Metabolism: The chemical processes which occur in cells of organisms which are necessary for the maintenance of life.

Micronutrients: The life-sustaining components in foods which are generally required in relatively small amounts but which may have a very significant effect on health.

Molecules: All of the structures in our bodies are made up of molecules which consist of atoms joined together in particular patterns.

Monounsaturated fatty acid: These have a chemical structure with only one double bond in their entire structure.

Nutrients: The components in foods which sustain life.

Obesity: This describes a state of being grossly overweight, and is associated with increased risks of illness and disease.

Oleic acid: This is a monounsaturated fatty acid. It is the predominant fat in olive oil and derives its name from the olive.

Oleocanthal: This is a specific polyphenol found in extra virgin olive oil which has antioxidant and anti-inflammatory properties.

Omega-3 fatty acid: This is a polyunsaturated fatty acid which the body is unable to manufacture for itself. It has bonds in the third position of the fatty acid molecule. The most common Omega-3 fatty acid is also known as alphalinolenic acid.

Omega-6 fatty acid: This is a polyunsaturated fatty acid which the body is unable to manufacture for itself. Its bonds are in the sixth position of the fatty acid molecule. The most common Omega-6 fat is called linoleic acid.

Omega-9 fatty acid: This is a monounsaturated fatty acid. It has the double-bond in the ninth position of the fatty acid molecule. The most common Omega-9 is also known as oleic acid.

Osteoarthritis: A condition characterised by painful and stiff joints, which may become swollen and cause disability.

Oxidative stress: This occurs when free radicals attack and damage cells in the body.

Palmitic acid: This is a saturated fatty acid which is thought to be one of the most harmful.

Parkinson's disease: A condition where a part of the brain becomes progressively damaged, having an effect particularly on movement, though which may also result in decline in memory, language and more general psychological and physical effects.

Peroxide: Peroxides are chemicals that are formed when fats break down as result of oxidation.

Phenol: This is a molecule of hydrogen and oxygen with a hexagonal structure. Some of the most complex chemicals found in our foods are made up of lots of phenols in various different combinations, therefore called polyphenols. Tyrosol, found in extra virgin olive oil is a good example.

Phenolic: See Phenols

Phyto-nutrients: Vitamins, minerals and anitoxidants carried in the coloured pigments of many plants. Also known as Phyto-chemicals.

Plaques: Plaque formation on the inner surface of blood vessel walls is part of a complex process involved in arteriosclerosis, eventually resulting in diseased arteries.

Platelets: Blood cells, the function of which is to promote the formation of clots. This is primarily designed to prevent haemorrhage when blood vessel walls are damaged.

Polyphenols: See Phenol.

Polyunsaturated fatty acid: These have a chemical structure with more than one double bond between the carbon atoms.

Pomace: This is the name given to the residue of olive flesh and stones that remains after the oil has been extracted.

Pro-inflammatory: Something which increases inflammation. This may describe the property of a chemical or a substance which has that effect.

Pyropheophytin: This substance is a natural product from the breakdown of green chlorophyll.

Pulses: Members of the legume family of plants, the edible seeds of which are dried as foods.

Rancidity: The effect of decomposition, especially of edible fats through oxidation, resulting in a foul taste and smell.

Redox: This is the name given to a balanced state of equilibrium in cells where any oxidative stress is balanced by our cells natural antioxidant capacity.

Rheumatoid arthritis: An autoimmune disease of joints characterised by inflammation, pain, swelling and stiffness especially, though not exclusively involving the joints of the hands and feet.

Saturated fatty acid: These have a chemical structure with no double bonds in their make up. All the carbon atoms are linked to hydrogen atoms.

Spectrophotometer: This is a machine which measures the absorption of UV light at specific wavelengths to detect levels of particular molecules. It relies on the principle that certain compounds have particular patterns of absorption or transmission of UV light.

Squalene: A specific hydrocarbon molecule found in the body and also in certain foods which has been the subject of research for its possible anti cancer effects.

Tamoxifen: This is a drug used to treat breast cancer.

Telomeres: These are protective caps on the stands of DNA which makes up our chromosomes. They get shorter every time a cell divides.

Thermogenesis: The production of heat.

Trans-fats: These are unsaturated fats which have undergone 'hydrogenation'. This is chemical process in which hydrogen is added to the original fat molecule.

Tri-glycerides: A fat which is comprised of three fatty acids attached to a molecule called glycerol.

Ulcerative colitis: This is a disease where bowel symptoms occur as a consequence of inflammation of the wall of the colon – the lower part of the gastrointestinal tract.

Vitamins: These are essential micronutrients which are needed for health and which the body is unable to manufacture for itself.

INDEX